EMS *Stress*

An Emergency Responder's Handbook For Living Well

EMS Stress

An Emergency Responder's Handbook For Living Well

Ray Shelton, Ph.D., EMT-CC and Jack Kelly, EMT

Foreword by Jeffrey T. Mitchell, Ph.D.

Acquisitions Editor . . . . .Rina Steinhauer

Developmental Editor . . . . .Brigitte Wilke

Editorial Assistant/Maryland . . . . .Melissa Blair

Editorial Assistant/California . . . . .Jennifer Delroy

Art/Production Manager . . . . .Ramona Higgins

Cover and Interior Design . . . . .The Jems Book Team

Illustrations . . . . .Arlette Ramphal

Photographs . . . . .Randall Lee (pp. 2, 26, 68, 104)
Cheryl Howlett (pp. 132, 134, 187,205)
Peter Escobedo (pp. 16, 20, 30, 37, 76, 113, 162, 188, 248)
Chris Weeks (pp. 194)
Heidi Maetzold (pp. 217)
Sharon Morine (pp. 222)
Harriet Wilcox (pp. 213)

The Jems Book Team:

Melissa Blair, Kathy Bush, Roberto Chávez, Rob Crippin, Elizabeth DiPinto, Jennifer Delroy, Ramona Higgins, Janene Long-Forman, Rina Steinhauer, and Harriet Wilcox

Library of Congress Catalog Card Number: 94-78604

Jems Communications is a subsidiary of
Mosby-Yearbook, Inc., a Times Mirror Company

P.O. Box 2789, Carlsbad, CA 92018
Tel: (619) 431-9797

ISBN: 0-8151-7512-4
Book Code Number: 24613
Jems Product Code: JP202

Table of Contents ———————————

Foreword

EMS Stress is a lighthouse in a world awash with demands, complications, egocentricity and greed. It is a book for the generous, self-giving kind of person who wears weary with so much concern for others. It is a book for the caretaker who needs a little guidance in caring for themselves.

Most emergency service personnel are as sophisticated and as highly trained in the technology of life saving as is humanly possible at this time in history. The fact is that almost all of the training is technological in nature and virtually none of it prepares people to manage their own response to human misery. Only a few books exist which address the needs of emergency services personnel in the care of themselves. This book is a welcome addition to the small library of texts designed to assist emergency personnel in surviving in a demanding job in a complicated world.

EMS Stress could serve as an owners manual for people who are involved in emergency work. It is about living and loving well. The book is filled with helpful hints for survival in the midst of chaos. If only a few of the suggestions are followed, emergency personnel would be much healthier and their relationships would be more fulfilling for all parties involved.

EMS Stress is not the usual stress management book! Few general stress books could claim the attention of the reader the way EMS Stress does. The writing flows easily. The chapters connect in a sensible manner and are filled with an exciting array of interesting information, good stories and practical stress management suggestions. Exciting photos and graphics pepper the entire text.

This book should be read by anyone who works in a people care profession which deals with pain and death and work pressure. It will serve as a foundation stone in maintaining happiness and health for those who touch the pain of so many others.

Jeff Mitchell, Ph.D.
September 1994

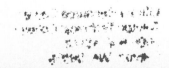

Acknowledgements ————————————————

The publisher wishes to acknowledge the invaluable
contributions of the reviewers of this book:

Linda B. Arters, B.A., EMT
Public Relations Consultant
  to the Emergency Services Industry
Chairman, Southwest Region CISM Network
Tempe, Arizona

Sarah A. Bohn, Ph.D.
Clinical Psychologist
Carlsbad, California

Mary F. Whiteside, Ph.D.
Associate Professor
Office of Medical Education
University of Texas Southwestern
  Medical Center at Dallas
Dallas, Texas

Preface

This book has been written for emergency responders by emergency responders. Both of the authors are EMTs with years of experience in the field. When we talk about the problems, frustrations, dangers and rewards of emergency response work, we are speaking from the lessons we've learned in our own lives.

We know what it's like: the tedious hours of training, the tones sounding at three in the morning, the rush of adrenaline, the chaos and confusion at a disaster scene, the bad feelings we get when we lose a patient, the good feelings that come from knowing we've saved a life or made a sick child smile.

In discussing EMS stress, we've included the stories and voices of real emergency responders—medics, police officers, firefighters, and nurses. We've compiled advice and information that applies to the real world, that makes sense in terms of our own lives and the lives of the emergency responders we've talked to.

Stress is no joke. It can be a serious, even life-threatening problem. The solutions we offer here can help you to deal with many types and degrees of stress. But sometimes a person finds himself in a difficult situation from which there seems to be no exit. Then it's important for you to recognize that stress is overwhelming your ability to cope. That's when you should seek help from a counselor or therapist. Don't delay. The help is out there waiting for you.

Stress can cause a wide variety of physical symptoms ranging from headaches and insomnia to chest pains and panic attacks. These symptoms are very real even if they are stress-related. Consult your physician at once if your symptoms indicate serious trouble. **Don't dismiss any symptom as "just stress."**

Finally, remember that we're all in this together. You can help your brothers and sisters in emergency service by passing on some of what you've learned in this book. If a solution works for you, maybe it will work for someone else. Some will welcome your advice, some will reject it. Your mission is to open doors for those suffering the effects of stress.

CHAPTER 1

Overview: Using This Handbook

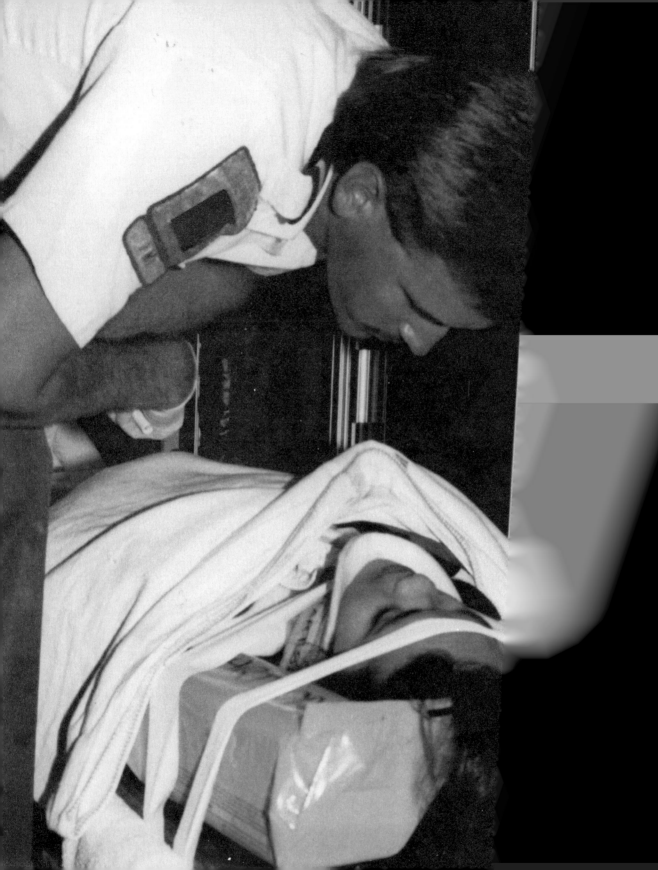

Overview

Is stress real? It's a question worth asking. Look out your window on a windy day. You don't see the wind. You see trees swaying, leaves fluttering, dust blowing. These are the effects of wind. Even though you don't see it, the wind is real. When you're fighting a brush fire in a gale, you know it's real.

What we call stress is the effect that events create on us. Just as you don't see the wind, you don't always see the stress in your life. What you see is the effect of the stress. It can take the form of illness, failed relationships, and difficulties on the job or at home.

Stress can come from all the events of your life. Marriage, the birth of a baby, even a vacation can be stressful. So can illness, job pressures, or powerful incidents in emergency service.

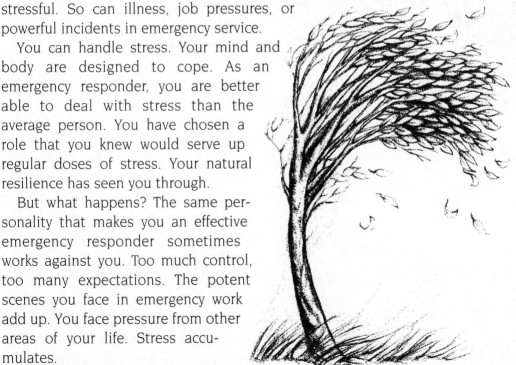

You can handle stress. Your mind and body are designed to cope. As an emergency responder, you are better able to deal with stress than the average person. You have chosen a role that you knew would serve up regular doses of stress. Your natural resilience has seen you through.

But what happens? The same personality that makes you an effective emergency responder sometimes works against you. Too much control, too many expectations. The potent scenes you face in emergency work add up. You face pressure from other areas of your life. Stress accumulates.

Stress is not bad; it's not good. It's simply a part of life. It will be with you as long as you live and will end the day you die.

Not the day you're promoted.

Not the day your children start school.

Not the day you retire.

Not the day you win a million in the lottery.

> **The question is not how to live without stress, but how to live with it.**

The question is not how to live without stress, but how to live with it.

Why Learn About Stress?

The reaction of some EMS people when they encounter the subject of stress is: *Why should I learn this*? I don't suffer from stress. I'm a calm person by nature. I can handle any stress the job brings my way. I've proven it.

In fact, there are several good reasons to learn about stress, even if you don't feel you are currently having trouble dealing with the stress you face:

1) Stress can overwhelm anybody. Many of us think we are immune from stress until it's too late. People work in emergency service for years and never have a problem handling the stress until one day when they find themselves in serious trouble. The truth is that no one is immune from stress problems. It may not have happened to you yet, but you have a long life ahead of you and you don't know what the future holds.

2) The time to learn stress management skills is now. It would be foolish to imagine that you could learn to do CPR on the way to a call. It's foolish to wait until you are under excessive stress to learn how to deal with it. Gaining a thorough knowledge of coping skills now will help you enormously when the crunch comes.

3) Prevention is better than cure. Many of the techniques discussed here are intended to ward off the effects of stress before they overwhelm you. Once you become

locked in a spiral of stress, it becomes much more difficult to get out of it.

4) Stress is insidious. It's important to be alert to the symptoms of stress even if you think you are coping adequately. It is not uncommon to be blindsided by a stress reaction when you least expect it.

5) Your colleagues will be facing stress. The people you work with may need assistance in dealing with stress. You can be the one to help them to cope with a critical incident or to alert them of the need to step back and deal with daily stress. But you must first develop the awareness and learn about the skills yourself.

Signing on for Stress

You know that stress is real. It's not just in your mind. It can affect your health, your job performance, your marriage, your life in general. Maybe you've seen the effects in your own life or in the lives of people close to you.

You know that stress is a part of emergency service. When you put on a uniform and clip a pager to your belt, you're signing on for stress. There's no way around it. The bad calls aren't the only source of stress. Emergency service puts physical demands on you, it cuts into your time, it can strain relationships with those you love, and it requires you to make adjustments in many areas of your life.

You know that stress can sneak up on you. You can't pin it down to one event. It's a combination of stresses in your emergency work and in your daily life that accumulate, wear you down, and finally do you in.

You know that there's no way to put an end to stress. Stress is a by-product of living, generated by both positive and negative events. Winning the lottery can be as stressful as a multi-casualty incident.

Winning the lottery can be as stressful as a multi-casualty incident.

When Tragedy Strikes

Sometimes questions arise in the discussion of stress management regarding the difference between "garden variety" stress and major life events like the death of a loved one. How can the two be compared? How can you think in the same terms about the stress of being caught in traffic and the stress of being told you have cancer?

Clearly, garden variety stress and major life event stress are vastly different things. But they do have elements in common. You have to deal with each type of incident and move on. A major event may permanently alter the quality of your life; but you must still find a way to cope and continue.

The tragic events of life await all of us. Learning how to handle the garden variety of stress successfully is the best way to prepare to manage much more serious forms of stress.

The tragic events of life await all of us. Learning how to handle garden variety stress successfully is the best way to prepare to manage much more serious forms of stress. You need to acquire and use the skills in advance so that you will be prepared when the time comes. The purpose of this book is to help you develop the type of coping techniques that apply to all forms of stress.

The Skills to Cope

There's no doubt that stress is responsible for the high rate of turnover in emergency service. But the good news is that you are uniquely qualified to handle the pressures that come with emergency service because you already have many of the necessary skills.

What have you learned in your training? To size up a situation under pressure. To keep your head even when chaos threatens. To act decisively in an emergency.

In many ways, stress is an emergency in your life. It's a situation, large or small, that requires action. Many of your emergency skills will apply. You need to survey the situation, to make an assessment. You need to keep things in perspective, decide on priorities, approach the situation with confidence. And you need to do something, to take the actions that bring the situation under control.

Some Sources of EMS Stress

Environment—cold, heat, noise

Time pressures

Emotional demands

Interpersonal conflicts

Paperwork

Desire for advancement

Perfectionism

Decision-making

Heavy workload

Physical danger

Red tape

Demands of patients

Threat of communicable disease

Rules and regulations

Training and drills

Boredom

Lack of recognition

Fatigue

Strain of lifting, carrying

Role ambiguity

Distraught bystanders

Uncertainty

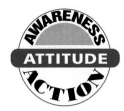

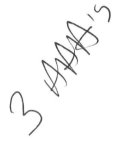

Awareness, Attitude, Action

Imagine you're a fire chief. You arrive on the scene of a major working structure fire. What's the first thing you do?

Awareness. You quickly step back and survey the whole scene. Are other structures in danger? Is there a tank of propane nearby? Are victims trapped inside?

Attitude. You are determined to bring the situation under control. You convey confidence and a calm sense of purpose to your people.

Action. You go to work and put out the fire. You address priority tasks first and proceed in a determined way toward your goal.

You will apply these same ideas to coping with stress.

Awareness

Roger was an EMT with more enthusiasm than experience. He arrived on the scene of a bad auto accident. The driver of the car was pinned inside. He was bleeding from a severe scalp laceration. Roger ran over to him. In his mind he was reviewing everything he'd learned in class about head wounds. As he reached out to help the injured man, he was knocked backward onto the ground, receiving second-degree burns to his hands and arms. In his haste, he hadn't noticed the power wires draped across the car's roof.

Roger didn't take the time to step back. He was gripped by tunnel vision. Every emergency responder has experienced it. We're so focused on what we're doing that we become oblivious of everything around us.

Awareness means being awake, being alert to the things going on in all aspects of your life. It's easy to spend a good part of your life daydreaming. When you're not aware, stress sneaks up on you. Stressful events themselves tend to distort your awareness. They draw your attention, causing you to lose sight of other important parts of your life.

> *Awareness means being awake, being alert to the things going on in all aspects of your life.*

It's possible to have a high tension wire draped across your life and not realize it's there. You have very shaky control of your emotions, fly off the handle at minor provocations. You're tired all the time, but you can't sleep. You suffer headaches, colds, problems with your digestion. People get on your nerves. The weight of the world is on your shoulders. And yet you're still telling yourself you have it all together, nothing's wrong.

Awareness means being alert for signs that stress has a hold on you. Ask yourself three questions:

How long has this been going on? An occasional bout of insomnia doesn't indicate a stress problem. But when it becomes habitual, it's time to assess yourself.

How bad is it? To argue with a colleague is one thing. To fly into a blind rage may indicate a serious stress problem.

Can I function? An inability to concentrate on your work or to get along with the people in your squad means that stress is taking over.

You know the value of assessment. It's the first thing you learn in EMT class. You can't provide the proper care without looking at everything from mechanism of injury to vital signs. In the same way, you can't get a handle on stress without first stepping back and becoming aware of the ways in which your life is out of balance.

Attitude

Awareness is about seeing. Attitude is about how we see. Consider the reaction of two EMTs when tones sound and the dispatcher announces a motor vehicle accident, person trapped. Martha has 15 years of experience. She moves quickly but deliberately. She makes sure she has all her equipment, takes time to fasten her seat belt. The adrenaline is flowing, but Martha takes a few deep breaths as she drives. She is mentally reviewing her skills. She sees herself successfully accomplishing whatever needs to be done.

Pete reacts to the same alarm in a different way. He runs out of the house, buttoning his shirt as he goes. He runs back for the turnout coat he forgot. His tires squeal as he backs out of his driveway. On the way, he starts imagining what he might find at the scene. His mouth goes dry. He's not sure he'll know what to do. He can see himself making mistakes. His own car practically skids off the road as he rounds a bend.

Martha and Pete are responding to the same stressful stimulus. What's the difference? Attitude—how they think about and react to the event. Two people can always face the same set of circumstances in entirely different ways:

▶ For one person, it's a disaster.
For the other, it's a minor obstacle.

▶ For one person, it's a crisis.
For the other, an opportunity.

▶ For one person, it's the end of the world.
For the other, a welcome challenge.

Question: Which person will suffer more stress? It's obvious. Pete's reaction to the alarm is the key to his stress. Stress is our reaction to events, not the events themselves.

Stress is our reaction to events, not the events themselves.

You took your EMT test and failed it by two points. The end of the world? A waste of all those hours? Or an opportunity to bone up on your weaknesses, study even harder, and become a better EMT than you would have been if you'd passed it the first time? It's a matter of perspective, attitude.

A great deal of stress results from the attitude that we're not in control of what is happening to us. In fact, many of the events in our lives are beyond our immediate control. But what we can control is how we react to events, our attitude toward them.

10

One EMT kept a card up near his desk with this message on it:

- *He didn't make me feel this way.*
- *She didn't make me feel this way.*
- *They didn't make me feel this way.*
- *It didn't make me feel this way.*
- *I chose to feel this way.*

Attitude means approaching life with confidence and determination. It means keeping a positive outlook. Why? Because the world is a rose garden? You know it's not. Because taking a positive view of life works—it helps you to deal with all the negatives that are bound to come your way.

Attitude means being able to step back from a situation and laugh. When emergency service people are called out, it's never to a party. It's always a scene of illness, injury, pain, or death. You have to counteract the negative by taking advantage of opportunities to laugh.

Given the things you see everyday, humor can be a life-saver. "There ain't much fun in medicine," someone once said, "but there's a heck of a lot of medicine in fun."

Action

As an emergency response person, you are action-oriented. You don't analyze auto accidents, contemplate fires, or theorize about illness. You act. You pull people out of cars, you put out real fires, you protect innocent people, you provide treatment that sometimes saves lives.

Your approach to stress should be to act, to do something. It's important to understand the mechanisms of stress, to be able to recognize its signs, and to be familiar with the ways it can affect your life. Awareness and attitude are crucial to controlling the effects of stress. But in the end, it's what you do that counts.

Action means having a plan and following through on it.
It means setting achievable goals.
It means starting from where you are, not where you wish you were.

Action is a key part of stress management because stress is really a summons to action. The stress reaction originates in an arousal, in the fight-or-flight reaction to a perceived danger.

Action is a way of taking control. If stress is causing you to become socially isolated, wishing for more friends won't work. You have to take specific steps to broaden your contacts, to keep in touch with people. If your stress is a result of never having enough time, sit down, determine how you use your time, eliminate low priority activities, and get yourself organized.

The concepts work together:

Awareness means recognizing when stress is becoming an issue in your life. It includes learning about where stress comes from and what it is doing to you.

Attitude means keeping things in perspective, taking responsibility, and deciding to survive.

Action means doing what's needed in order to handle the stress you will face and its effects on your life.

Options –
What I can change.
Accept what I can't.

The 10 Commandments of Stress Management

The following "10 Commandments" summarize some of the best techniques for coping with the stress in your life. For now, think about what they might mean and how they might apply to your own life and emergency work. You will find each of them identified by the clipboard symbol and explained as you proceed through the text.

THE 10 COMMANDMENTS
OF STRESS MANAGEMENT

I   Maintain a Life Away From Emergency Service

II   Have the Strength to Let Go

III Don't Be Afraid to Seek the Help of a Professional

IV   Don't Fight Change, Use it to Your Advantage

V   Nourish Your Mind As Well As Your Body

VI   Start From Where You Are—Don't Worry About the Past

VII Talk About What's Bothering You

VIII Don't Sweat the Small Stuff

IX   Take Time to Laugh

X   Set Goals to Give Your Life Purpose and Adventure

CHAPTER 2

The Stress of Daily Life

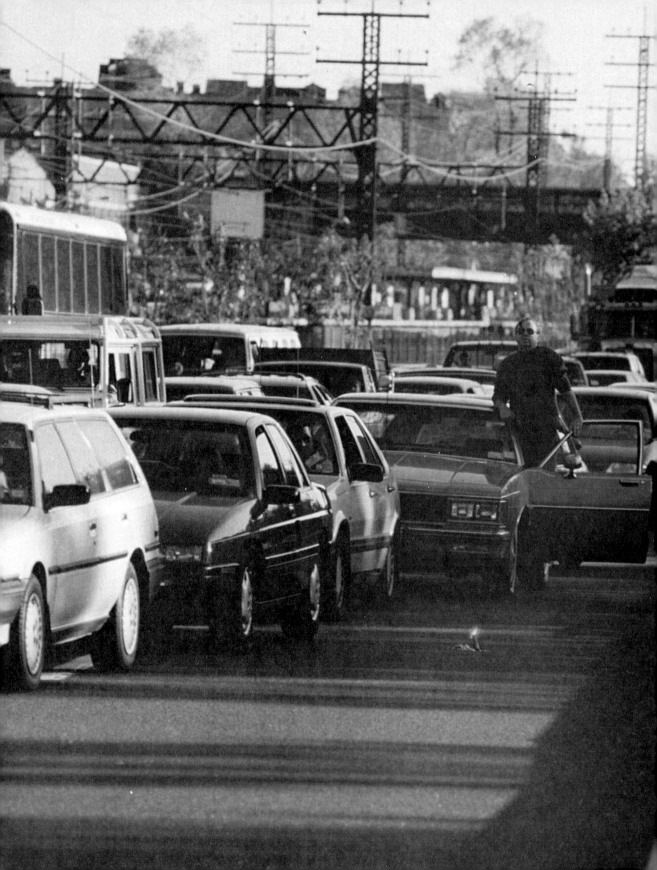

The Stress of Daily Life

"I had it all together. Things were going good in my life. We'd just moved into our house. It needed some repairs and I found myself staying up at night trying to get everything fixed up the way we wanted it.

"About the same time we closed on the house, I was elected captain of my ambulance company. Now, instead of spending one night a week at the station, I was there almost five nights in a row. There was always another administrative detail to take care of. Plus I felt pressured to make more calls, to set an example.

"A few months later, I started my EMT refresher course. That cut into my time. I began to have trouble getting out of bed in the morning. I couldn't concentrate on my job. For the first time in seven years I received a bad performance review.

"My wife and I argued about the house—I still hadn't finished the work on it. Days would go by, it seemed like, and I wouldn't have a chance to spend time with my baby daughter. Around this time we had a couple of bad calls—a man of 50 in cardiac arrest, an accident where the patient went into shock and died in the hospital. No worse than usual, but the kind of things that stick with you.

"I know it didn't happen overnight, but I never saw it coming. Suddenly I didn't have it all together. My marriage was shaky, I had problems at work, and the board of directors at my ambulance company suggested I take a leave of absence. I had too many balls in the air and they were starting to drop.

"My wife had been telling me to slow down, and I just hadn't heard her. I thought I was just busy, but now I realize I'd lost the ability to relax and let go. How could I relax? I had the weight of the world on my shoulders—I felt that if I relaxed I'd be crushed."

What is Stress?

This Emergency Medical Technician's story will sound familiar to anyone who has devoted time to emergency service. Emergency service provides innumerable instances of stress: fatal car crashes, children dying, multi-casualty incidents.

But stress is a much broader concept than these obvious examples would suggest. The stress that you have to cope with will come from all the areas of your life, not just from emergencies. It may originate in a single incident, or it may result from an accumulation of small events. It may affect you right away, or weeks, months, or years later.

The word stress can be defined in several ways. Stress is any response to the events of our lives. Stress is pressure from outside that makes us feel tense inside. Stress is a nonspecific response of the body to demands put on it.

Stress happens inside you. A stressor is the event in the world that you are reacting to. Your mind is the powerful instrument that mediates between the stressors you encounter and the stress reactions that you undergo.

stress In its simplest form, stress is a reaction in your mind and body to an event in the outside world that alarms or arouses you.

——STRESS IS——

Stress is a response to a perceived threat, challenge, or life change.

Stress is a physical and psychological response to any demand.

Stress is a state of psychological and physical arousal.

Balance

One of the important lessons you learned when becoming an EMT was to consider the entire patient rather than to focus only on an obvious injury. The nightmare of every EMT is to deliver a patient to the hospital, his broken arm splinted in textbook fashion, only to realize that he's going into hypovolemic shock from an abdominal hemorrhage you never bothered to assess for.

A similar principle applies to stress. Don't just focus on the immediate cause. Someone makes a suggestion about how you could have handled a call. The comment enrages you, you blow up, the discussion turns into a shouting match. Is the person's criticism the cause of your stress? Probably not. Maybe it's a difficult call you went on a week ago. Maybe it's pressure you've been under at work, all accumulating to a flash point.

Stress problems do not call for Band-Aid solutions. If you regularly suffer insomnia, the answer is not a sleeping pill. You need to look at yourself as a total person. You have a number of facets to your life—physical, emotional, social. When problems hit one area, your whole being tends to go out of alignment. The best ways of coping with stress consider all areas of your total person.

Wellness

Health is not a condition, it's a direction. Some things move us toward well-being: eating right, exercising, taking time to relax, engaging in recreational activities, spending time with people we like. These activities counteract the forces that push us the other way: physical strains, overwork, anger, isolation, excessive drinking.

Wellness means regularly taking action to move yourself toward the positive end of the spectrum of health. To embrace the idea of wellness is your best defense against stress.

Wellness means regularly taking action to move yourself toward the positive end of the spectrum of health.

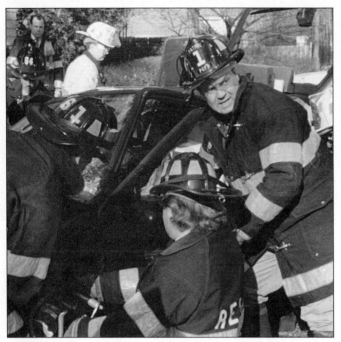

Every emergency responder endures physical, emotional, and mental burdens that drag that person toward illness. To leap out of a warm bed on a winter night and respond to a bad accident takes something out of you. To have someone die while you work to save them carries an emotional toll. To be required to learn and remember everything that an EMT has to know, and realize that someone's life may depend on it, is a heavy responsibility.

Therefore, every emergency responder needs to do things that promote wellness. You can't stand still. If you're not actively fighting the adverse effects of stress, stress will get the better of you sooner or later. Too many emergency responders have learned that from experience.

Taking Time for Yourself

A 70-year-old ex-fire chief talked to some young members after a meeting. Someone asked him how he'd lasted so long.

"The best piece of advice I can give you," he said, "is don't ever let the fire service become your entire life. In the 52 years I was in active service, I always made sure I had a balance in my life. I made time for my wife, enjoyed my kids, and made sure we spent time together as a family. I never got out of bed when I was sick just to make a call. And I didn't worry about it.

"Anything you do in your life, no matter how much you enjoy it, do it all the time and you'll end up hating it. When you're out there, be the best you can. But when you're away from it, learn to leave it alone. Take care of yourself and your family first. If you can do that, you may be giving this same advice to some rookie 50 years from now."

I   Maintain a Life Away From Emergency Service

It's important to have a full life away from EMS. That is what will sustain you when stress hits. Too many of us fall into a pattern where emergency service becomes all-consuming. The ambulance station becomes a second home, our social activities involve only other squad members, we read emergency medical journals, talk about EMS, eat and sleep EMS.

Every one of us needs to spend time with friends who have no connection to emergency service, to find rewarding and absorbing activities that recharge our batteries.

Take time to play. EMS work is always serious, sometimes grim. For one advanced EMT, it's model trains. *"When I'm playing with my trains, I'm not thinking about EMS or about work," he says. "I'm having fun. It's a totally different world. I can let go of the pressures of life, forget the bad call I've been on. This hobby keeps my head together and lets me do my job better."*

The Power of the Mind

Your best weapon for fighting stress is right between your ears. Changing the way you think about stress is an important step toward neutralizing it. There are many ways to think yourself through a stressful situation:

Look at it in perspective. Keep an eye on the big picture, on what's really important.

Put aside the negative. By learning to shut off nagging doubts and worries, you can improve your mental clarity and alleviate many instances of stress.

Look at the facts. Knowledge defuses stress. Think how much more fearful and apprehensive you would have felt if you had encountered an auto accident before becoming an EMT.

A Family Matter

This book is not just for you. Most of us have a spouse or someone who is special to us. We have family, maybe children. It's important, as you learn about stress, to include the people closest to you in your solutions.

One of the most precious things at risk for EMS people is relationships. The simple fact is, emergency service puts demands on our time, our attention, our emotional reserves. It may lead us to neglect those closest to us. It can cause conflict, arguments, or resentment. One of the most common and most serious consequences of EMS stress is isolation. We withdraw, and soon problems at home begin to compound the stresses we encounter in our emergency work.

> *One of the most precious things at risk for EMS people is relationships.*

The way to avoid this conflict is to make sure your loved ones understand just as much as you do about the stresses and demands of emergency work. That doesn't mean describing the grisly scenes you encounter in the field or sharing the details of every call. It does mean talking about how you feel, about how EMS work affects you. It means letting that person comfort you when you need to be comforted—and we all do at times. It means reserving some time together no matter how busy you both are. It means communicating, sharing, and trusting each other.

It's a good idea, as you proceed through the book, to take the time to talk over with your significant other many of the issues raised along the way. That person can often be your most valuable resource when it comes to winning the battle against stress.

SUMMARY

- When you become involved in emergency service, stressful events become a regular part of your life.
- The best way to cope with day-to-day stress is through the AAA approach introduced in Chapter 1:

Awareness, Attitude, Action

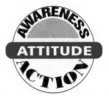

- The stress of daily life is as important to consider as is the stress of critical incidents.

  Balance is a key concept in handling stress.

  Take time for yourself.
  Maintain a full life away from your emergency work.
  Use the power of your mind to combat the effects of stress.
  Make stress management a family matter, include those close to you.

For Further Thought

1. Try applying the concepts of awareness, attitude, and action to some typical stress scenarios.

   For example, Bob tries to make every call at his busy volunteer rescue squad. He's tired all the time, isn't performing well at work, and feels pressured.

   Awareness—Bob has to step back and see that his EMS work is cutting into time he should reserve for himself.

   Attitude—He needs to recognize that the squad can function without him some of the time.

   Action—Bob selects certain time slots that he reserves for himself and his family by turning off his pager.

Think about these situations using the AAA approach:

   Diane's husband can't understand why she won't talk about the things that happen on her rescue calls. She says he wouldn't understand. It's gotten to be a point of contention between them.

Ted went out on a very bad call a month ago. A 5-year-old boy drowned in a quarry; Ted did CPR on him for half an hour. Now he can't get the image of the incident out of his mind. He's having trouble sleeping.

Dan has been involved in EMS for almost 20 years. He has none of the spark he had when he started. He spends much of his time in front of the television. Everything seems like a chore to him.

2. Think of the last time you were close to being overwhelmed by stress. How might awareness, attitude, and action have helped you to deal with that situation?

3. What are three EMS-related sources of stress that are affecting you today? What are some other sources of stress in your life?

4. What made you get involved in EMS in the first place? Do you remember what you expected when you entered the field?

5. Can you think of an example in which a lack of awareness added to your stress?

6. Small things often cause us stress because they appear to be big things at the time. Can you think of a time in which a little perspective would have prevented a lot of stress?

7. Sometimes the things that would help you to better handle stress—going out to dinner with your spouse, getting together with a friend whose company you enjoy—end up far down on your list of priorities. Make a short list of things you want to do and then do them—sooner rather than later.

CHAPTER 3

Stress and the Emergency Responder

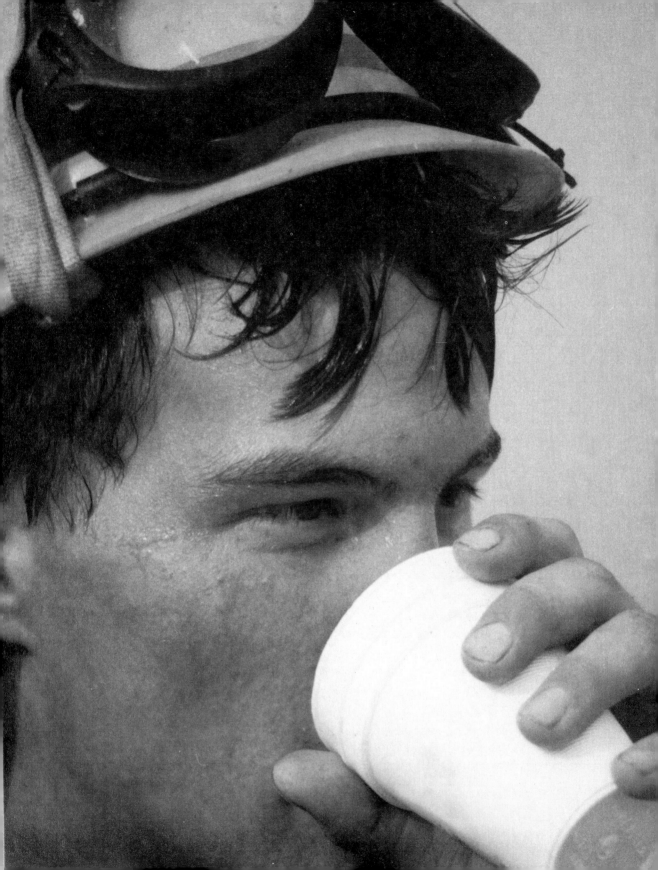

Stress and the Emergency Responder

A few days after a plane crash involving numerous casualties, one of the rescuers told this story to a roomful of his fellow emergency responders:

"I have been a firefighter for 25 years. For the past 10 years, I have been a captain in one of the busiest engine companies in the city. I have also been a volunteer firefighter near my home for 15 years. I'm married. I have never cried in front of my wife in the 28 years we've been together. Until now.

"I arrived at the crash site at 10:04 p.m. I stayed on the scene until six in the morning. It was not the worst scene I have responded to in my years of service. But it was bad. Kids were hurt. Kids were dead. That's what I remember most.

"I did the usual rescue thing. I assisted with extrication. I carried out bodies.

"When I got home, I remember sitting on my bed, leaning over to take off my shoes. Out of the corner of my eye I saw the picture of my three sons on the night table.

"I began to weep. I couldn't stop. My wife heard me, came into the room. She sat down on the bed beside me, put her arms around me, held me, and let me cry. I remember her saying, 'It's OK. I'm here. Let it go.'

"What I want to say to all of you is this: During those 28 years of marriage, I would never allow myself to show emotion to my family. I always had to be the tough guy. I remember fighting back tears at my mom's funeral. Why? So my kids wouldn't think I was weak.

"But at that moment, sitting on my bed, the emotion of what I had been seeing all night long hit me like a ton of bricks. So many kids. It didn't seem right. I guess I thought about how I would feel if it were my children.

"When I finished crying, my wife and I sat at the kitchen table and talked for an hour about the crash. In all my years of service, I never did anything like that. I always thought that she couldn't stand to hear about the bad calls, the death.

"Hey, guys, I can't begin to tell you why I wouldn't cry all those years. I think you understand why. And I tell you, as my brothers: I don't think I will ever be afraid to show my emotions again."

It's a story we can all identify with. For years, this man struggled with a conflict. He was a strong man. His strength made him an excellent firefighter and helped him to survive. It let him stare death in the face, help others, and save lives.

At the same time, his strength worked against him. It isolated him, made him take on burdens that he could have and should have shared. It left him in the grip of stress.

What Makes You Breaks You

"My friends and family can't understand why I like this stuff," was how a paramedic put it.

Can't understand why we want to be called out of bed at four o'clock on a winter morning to aid the sick and injured, to fight fires, to manage an accident scene. Can't understand why we want to deal with people who are injured, or violent, or dead. Can't understand, in the end, why we want to see and experience the things that we all do see—the serious things, the horrible things.

Emergency response work requires a special person, and a special personality. There is something special about those who are attracted to this work, something special about those who excel in it.

But it's important to note: The very traits that make you become an emergency responder can work against you. The traits that make you successful out in the field can undermine you in your life. The traits that make you, break you.

That's why it's important to begin your approach to stress by asking: Who am I?

Are You Susceptible To Stress?

No one is immune from the ill effects of stress. Some people, because of their personalities, are more susceptible than others.

In order to informally evaluate your susceptibility to stress, answer the following questions Yes or No:

1. I tend to be meticulous and pay attention to detail.

2. It's important what other people think of me.

3. Ideas and worries often come into my head again and again.

4. I am quick to take responsibility for the things that happen around me.

5. I can't keep myself from getting nervous at times.

6. I often feel lonely.

7. I worry about not being able to handle situations.

8. I have trouble sleeping when something is upsetting me.

9. I'm often critical of myself or others.

10. I become bored easily.

11. I often think of myself in a negative light.

12. I'm easily distracted.

13. I sometimes feel powerless to control things in my life.

14. I often feel isolated from other people.

15. I worry about losing emotional control.

If you answer yes to more than seven or eight of these items, it's important for you to take special care to guard against overload and burnout.

"I'm in Control"

Almost by definition, an emergency responder is a person with an aptitude for control. You walk into chaos: a

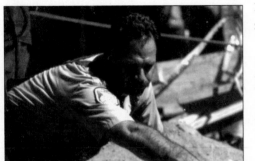

motor vehicle accident, a raging fire, a scene of sudden death. You bring order.

You control yourself when everyone around you is going berserk. You put your feelings aside and keep your head.

You control other people. You have a "command presence." Your attitude inspires victims and bystanders to begin to get a grip on themselves.

You control situations. You bring a fire under control. You stabilize the condition of a trauma patient. You control traffic.

Control is good. Control is your job.

But control can break you. It begins when you fall victim to **The Superhuman Myth:** I can do it all. I'm always in control. Nothing fazes me, nothing bothers me, nothing shakes me. I divide my life into compartments. What happens out in the streets, in the field, doesn't touch the other parts of my life. I'm immune. I don't burden my family or friends with it—they wouldn't understand anyway.

I don't cry, ever. Tears mean weakness and I'm strong. Nobody will see that I'm sometimes upset or sometimes afraid. Nobody will see my fears. Nobody will see my tears. Nobody—nobody will ever call me soft.

That's the myth. What's the reality?

You're human. What happens in the field does have an effect on you. It hits you hard, whether you show it or not. It touches parts of your life far removed from your emergency service.

The reality is: The tears are there whether you let them flow or not. Given the things you see, it's only natural. You're human.

But the firefighter who could not cry is all of us. We all find it hard to let go; we all try to control ourselves. We keep gritting our teeth when it's better to let go, when it's absolutely necessary to let go.

The tears are there whether you let them flow or not.

Tears are human. Weeping puts us in touch with our humanity and with ourselves. The important message that this firefighter learned was that you don't have to be in control all the time. That it's OK not to be OK.

II   Have the Strength to Let Go

The urge to control can bring us stress in other ways. Events and situations can't always be controlled. A volunteer EMT who responded to a bad auto accident said,

"We did everything by the book. The extrication went like clockwork. The patient was talking to me. I thought we'd done everything right. But on the way to the hospital he went out on us. We bagged him, did CPR. He died. It was frustrating to feel so useless. My image of myself was shattered by this experience."

Reality always has the last word. Sometimes it's hard to face that fact.

The ability to control other people, to direct them, calm them, is another asset of the emergency response personality. But again, it can create stress.

Have you ever taken your command presence home with you? Have you ever found yourself ordering around family members or friends? Do you find it hard to live and let live? Control can mean conflict. Conflict brings stress.

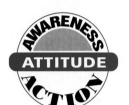

Awareness—

Be aware of the times when you can and should give up control. Recognize that letting go sometimes requires as much strength as holding in.

Attitude—

"Sometimes it's good to be in control, and sometimes it's good to express my feelings. I have the strength to let go."

Action—

1. Talk over with your colleagues the things that happen to you in emergency service. Sit down after a call or a few days later. Talk about how you felt as well as about what happened.
2. Get in the habit of regularly sharing your feelings with your spouse or someone close to you.

"I've Got High Hopes"

As an emergency responder you are probably an incurable optimist. You expect to make a difference. You see disaster, injury, death, and the next day you are out there doing your job, confident that you can save a life, help the sick.

The job you do is impossible without a high level of expectation. You're a planner. You anticipate. You aim high.

Expectations make you, expectations can break you. A good example is the police officer who wanted to better serve the community by gaining advance EMT certification and serving on a police ambulance:

"I'd already received basic EMT training on my own time. I was highly motivated. I sailed through the course and graduated with an average in the high 90's. My skills were textbook. I was assigned to the Emergency Ambulance Bureau. I expected to save lives.

"On my first ambulance call as an Advanced EMT, I responded to an 82-year-old male in cardiac arrest. This patient had a 15-year history of heart disease. Resuscitation efforts failed. My expectations were being challenged.

"Twenty-four hours later, I responded to a call for an electrocution. While using an electric drill in a do-it-yourself project, the man grabbed a water pipe. His wife found him later—he died.

"A week went by. A call came in for a child struck by a truck. On arrival, I found that a 7-year-old girl had ridden her bike into the path of a fully loaded, tandem-wheel dump truck. Extrication took 15 minutes. The girl died from mass trauma on the way to the hospital.

"I had come face to face with reality. My expectation—'I save lives'—suddenly collapsed. The fact that none of the lives could have been saved, even with intensive care on the scene, didn't matter. All that mattered to me were my expectations.

"On my next tour of duty, I ripped my Advanced EMT card in half, handed it to my commanding officer, and requested return to routine police patrol. I remember saying, 'No one will ever die on me again. I've had enough.'"

This officer was done in by another myth common among emergency responders—**The Superman Myth:**

- Faster than a speeding bullet, more powerful than a locomotive. Sound familiar?

- I can do the impossible. The odds against me don't matter. Every call will have a positive result. I'll never make a mistake. I'll never encounter a situation I can't handle. I'll never fail.

- I'm indestructible. Pain? Forget it. The accident, the injury will always happen to somebody else. I can work double shifts. I can lift any load. I can work a fire scene indefinitely.

What's the reality? **You aren't Superman. You have limits—we all do.** We can be injured, we feel pain. Not all of our patients will live. Some die. Some die in our presence. That's a fact. The most we can ever do is to do our best.

The downside of high expectations is frustration and disappointment. We expect thanks—sometimes we get sued. We expect to help people—sometimes they die on us. Failure is part of life. If you lack the flexibility to accept failure, the clash between your expectations and reality will generate stress.

The solution is to go easy on yourself. When you're tired, emotionally drained, or not feeling up to par, ease off. Step back from your emergency work.

Focus on your achievements instead of your failures. There are many small victories in EMS: you succeed in making a child smile, you ease an accident victim back from the edge of panic. Give yourself credit.

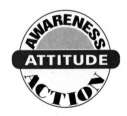

Awareness—

Think over the reasons why you first became involved in emergency work. Were some of your expectations unrealistic?

Attitude—

"I'm human. I do my best, but I can't expect everything to go my way all the time. I realize that I have limits."

Action—

1. Recognizing that no one can be good at everything, make a short list of your strengths and weaknesses.
2. Write down three recent achievements in your EMS work, no matter how small.

"I Can Still See It"

We are all familiar with the imprint of horror. A firefighter told this story:

"A commercial jetliner was landing in a thunderstorm on runway 22-Left at Kennedy Airport when the plane dropped 200 feet, crashed near the Rockaway Turnpike, and broke apart.

"It was an ugly crash. Burned bodies were scattered over the runway. The medical examiner's people gave me rubber gloves and told me to collect body parts—tag and bag anything that appeared human.

"I had been doing this for a couple hours. I was becoming depressed; it was time to take a break. I walked 75 yards away from the impact to where three city firemen and two emergency service police officers were also getting a breath of air.

"I lit a cigarette, began talking. When I shifted my foot, the ground didn't feel right. I moved my foot and looked down. I was standing on a human hand. I know it was a left hand because I clearly saw the wedding band. I tossed away the cigarette, put my gloves on, tagged the hand, put it in a bag.

"To this day, 20 years after the event, when I see a wedding band on a man's hand, I can tell you the names of those three firefighters and those two cops. I'd never met them before, haven't seen them since. I can smell that air, hear those sounds. But ask me what I had for dinner two nights ago, I doubt if I could tell you."

Attention to detail is good. In an emergency, your attention is cranked up. Details don't just register, they burn into your brain. You focus on the right things: mechanism of injury, hazards at the scene, a patient's vital signs.

Attention to detail can also break you. Events from years ago come back to you in technicolor. Vivid details haunt you.

It's important to recognize that these images, the vivid flashbacks and the intense feelings that go with them, are normal.

It doesn't have to be as graphic as a human hand. One EMT performed CPR on a male of 70. At the scene was a younger man. The patient did not survive. On the way home, the EMT heard in his mind three words that the young man had spoken, very quietly, during the crisis. "Come on, Dad." That tiny detail—and the lifetime of love it implied—was imprinted in the EMT's brain and evoked strong emotion years later.

Imprints can create stress. We become obsessed with charged memories. Images—a wedding band—become hot buttons. We are too easily thrown back into situations of extreme stress.

The solution is to talk about it. Mention it to your colleagues. If you cling to an image you give it power. Even an informal chat on the way back from an incident can help to neutralize this source of stress.

It's important to recognize that these images, the vivid flashbacks and the intense feelings that go with them, are normal. Everyone who is involved in emergency service experiences them.

Awareness—

- Am I obsessed by thoughts of things that have happened on calls?
- Do I avoid talking about these images so others won't think I'm crazy?

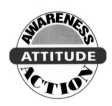

Attitude—

"The images and flashbacks that I have following intense episodes are completely normal. I don't mind talking about them."

Action—

1. Talk about any experience or image that stays with you. Get together with a colleague or close friend and describe what you saw.

2. When you come home after a call, write down details that stick in your mind or that bother you. This will serve to defuse them and help you to put them aside.

3. Following a critical incident, participate in one of the debriefing sessions that are commonly offered today. Even if you are not feeling troubled at the moment, the debriefing can head off problems that might develop later.

"I Love Action"

The alarm goes off. Tones sound. A call comes over the radio. The siren wails. Emergency lights flash. Your heart races. You know the feeling.

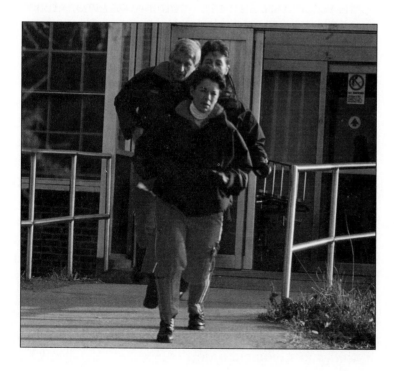

Let's face it, we're all "trauma junkies." We love action. We love that rush of adrenaline. Emergencies give us a charge. Action makes us. If we didn't like to ride that wave of excitement, we wouldn't have gone into this line of work.

Emergency response work really is exciting. It's always a challenge. It provides tremendous satisfaction. But life is not filled with disasters. Even in the busiest fire district, there's plenty of time between emergencies.

In fact, there's a whole other side to emergency work: the waiting, the paperwork, the meetings and classes and drills, the practice, recertification, false alarms, equipment reviews, seminars, deadly routine. But if you're "addicted" to that adrenaline rush, too long a time between exciting calls can make you nervous—you go through a kind of withdrawal.

Sometimes our need for action and risk makes it hard to accept routine. A new police officer said, "I thought police work was exciting. The highlight of my day is putting out the school stop sign each morning. How many times can I ride around the sector chasing barking dogs and looking for lost bikes?"

He was so disillusioned he was considering going back to his old job: fixing home appliances.

You can find a better balance if you don't depend on emergency work for all the action in your life. Find hobbies that excite you and fill your need for action. Physical activities are good. Take up ballet dancing or softball or skiing. Sky dive, ride a motorcycle, or climb mountains if that's where your inclinations lead. You might get a charge from community theater or sailing.

Be careful, though, to weigh the risks you take. Remember, you're not Superman. Don't forget to put on your parachute.

In order to keep the time between calls from weighing on you, vary your routine. Don't march through every day in a lockstep pattern. Take a different route to work. Do things in a different order.

Awareness—

- Am I frequently bored by the routine tasks connected with emergency work?
- Do I get "antsy" if too much time goes by between calls?
- In the excitement of a call do I take unnecessary risks, such as driving at high speeds?

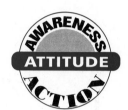

Attitude—

"I use the adrenaline rush to energize me and make me more alert, but I don't let it overwhelm me. I have activities away from emergency service that I find exciting."

Action—

1. List all the active or exciting things you've done in the past month. Are almost all of them connected with your emergency work? If so, regular participation in sports or other activities could be an important way for you to fight stress.

2. Make routine interesting: Turn a drill into a competition. Transform drudgery into a work party.

3. Don't let your taste for action overwhelm you. When the alarm sounds, get in the habit of taking a couple of deep breaths.

The Case of the Saber-Toothed Tiger

A story is often told to illustrate the origins of the stress response. Imagine you're living 10,000 years ago. You're walking home. You've had a good day. You've caught a few fish for your dinner. You're happy. This is before taxes, remember.

You hear a noise behind you. You're curious. What is it? Coming down the path is a saber-toothed tiger. That tiger is very interested in having you for his dinner.

Your body goes into overdrive. It's a reflex. Adrenaline floods your system. You're suddenly pumped up.

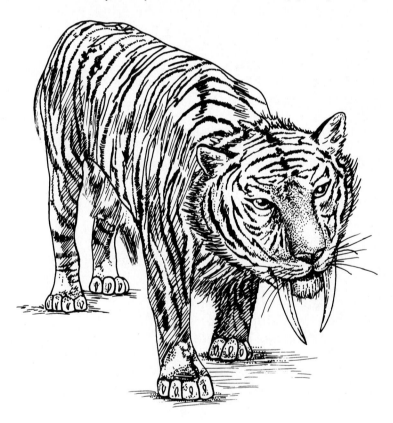

Your body is ready to wrestle with that tiger, or to run away. Of course, you're no fool—you run.

You run faster than you've ever run in your life. You sprint back to your cave. You make it inside to safety just ahead of the tiger.

When you've had a chance to catch your breath, you relax by the fire and tell the tale to your family and friends. Maybe you exaggerate a little for effect.

The point is, you're still that cave man today. Our bodies, our reflexes, haven't changed much in 10,000 years. And those reflexes can still be useful.

Let's say you're out walking today, only instead of a jungle path, it's the parking lot at the mall. You're alone. It's dark. A couple of guys are following you. You speed up. They speed up. You cut over an aisle. They cut over an aisle. Your heart starts to pound. They're closing in.

But now you're at your car. You jump in. Lock the door. Start the engine. Drive away. You've faced a real danger. Your arousal has worked the way it was designed—to help you avoid harm.

These days we face more paper tigers than we do real tigers. Paper tigers are the problems that arise when there's no cave to run to. Your arousal system kicks in, but there's nothing you can do to release the arousal.

Your fight-or-flight reaction gets turned on by things you can't fight. Usually you can't run away either. Paper tigers. Maybe it's an ornery boss at work. A demanding client. A bill you find in your mailbox. A misunderstanding with your wife. A traffic jam. Could be anything, or a combination of things.

Your body primes itself to act. But no physical action is needed. You don't spend your energy running, so you don't end up relaxed by the fire. The result is this thing called stress.

STRESS
The Body'

I n some ways, the physiological mechanisms that actually produce the stress reaction are like a 9-1-1 system for the body.

The cerebral cortex of the brain is the communication center, which receives and processes information about what is happening in your environment. Usually that information is routine. Occasionally it is alarming.

Cerebral Cortex

The limbic system of the brain can be compared to the dispatcher who takes the calls. This system makes the decision that classifies the information as an emergency requiring action.

The hypothalamus, farther down in the brain, is like the alarm system itself. This regulator of the body's chemistry sends its message down the sympathetic nervous system that controls the body's physiology. The alarm goes out in the form of epinephrine or adrenaline, which is secreted by the adrenal glands that ride on top of the kidneys.

Just as you heighten your awareness and prepare to take action when you hear an alarm sound, various systems of your body prepare for

Hypothalamus

action in response to the adrenaline alarm. Heart and respiratory rates increase. Muscles tense. Blood pressure goes up. The brain becomes more alert. The liver increases the

-1-1 *System*

blood glucose level. Other chemical changes take place that prepare you to fight or to run away.

The body can dissipate most of the effects of stress as it takes appropriate actions to deal with whatever caused the alarm. Once the source of arousal is gone, the brain

Limbic System

cancels the alarm through the parasympathetic nervous system. The body produces the chemical acetylcholine, which neutralizes the effects of the adrenaline. But if dissipation is not possible, or if the alarms come too frequently, the body remains in a state of partial alert all the time, and stress becomes a problem. It's a little like an ambulance squad that's overworked with too many calls, or that responds to a string of false alarms.

Sources of Stress

Where does your stress come from? When you think about this question, your mind immediately turns to the powerful, emotional scenes of your emergency work. But that is only one source. To assess your vulnerability to overload, you need to look at all sources of stress in your life.

The Boss

Who's the boss in your life? Most would say, my supervisor, the person who gives me orders at work.

But that's not your only boss. Your boss is anyone who expects you to perform. For emergency responders, anybody who picks up a phone and calls for help is your boss. And you know what demanding bosses they can be.

Your family is your boss. They expect you to provide an income, the roof over their heads, food on the table, and clean laundry.

A boss is always a source of stress. A boss can give you recognition—or fail to give it. A boss can threaten. A boss can criticize, sometimes without justification. A boss has control over a certain part of your autonomy.

stressor An event in the world that gives rise to a stress reaction inside you.

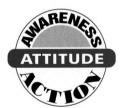

Awareness—

Who are your bosses? Make a list of them.

Attitude—

"My boss doesn't make me experience stress. I have control over what I feel."

Action—

Communicate. Whenever you can, clarify what it is your boss expects from you.

Deadlines

Are you wearing a watch? Most likely you are. You have a calendar on the wall, a planning book full of appointments and deadlines.

In emergencies, time suddenly turns into a life-and-death concern. You've learned about the "golden hour" for getting a trauma patient to the hospital. In CPR class you've learned about the four to six minutes that separate clinical and biological death.

If you had unlimited time, you would have no stress. But you are always pressured to get things done "on time." And when time is short, you are forced to make difficult decisions about priorities. Time pressures, deadlines, heavy workloads, all add to stress.

Awareness—

Why are you often in a hurry? What are your time pressures?

Attitude—

"I can bring my schedule under control. It's up to me to establish my priorities."

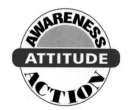

Action—

1. Break up deadlines. If you have a big project due in a month, divide it into four parts and finish one part each week. Learn to say no.
2. Examine all the little things that waste your time.

The Job

We would all like to look forward to our jobs every day, but for most of us, the job is a powerful source of stress.

One firefighter/EMT who worked in a very busy urban station reported becoming depressed two to three hours before reporting for his tour. He said that he was tired of endless scenes of death and destruction. He lay awake at night thinking about his job. Even during his days off he remained tense. The job was affecting his entire life.

Connected with the job are such stress-related issues as advancement, the need to go through training, and stressful working conditions. For those who work in emergency service on a volunteer basis, EMS work may cause conflicts with their regular jobs. It's hard to go put in a day's work if you've spent four hours at an accident scene in the middle of the night.

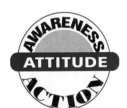

Awareness—

What is your job doing to you? Does it bore you? Do you have trouble getting along with co-workers?

Attitude—

"My job is important, but I am not my job. I have a life."

Action—

1. Learn a new skill that increases your perspective and opportunities in relation to your job.
2. Write down the goals you have for yourself at work.

Money

Debts. Bills. Credit cards. Mortgages. College finances. Medical expenses. Car payments. Money means stress. You struggle to meet today's obligations; you worry about the funds you will need tomorrow.

Money can push you over the edge. One young EMS worker said, "I found I had to take on two part-time jobs to support my family. After a day on the ambulance I worked a second job from 6 p.m. until 2 a.m. On weekends I covered extra shift at my regular job. I kept it up for three months before being hospitalized for exhaustion."

Money is really a symbol for security. A lack of security, one of our most basic needs, is a very potent source of stress.

Awareness—

Look at the financial facts of life. What's coming in and where is it going out?

Attitude—

"I don't need to be rich. I can make ends meet if I'm smart about it."

Action—

Draw up a realistic budget and stick to it. Consolidate debts. Keep track of where your money goes.

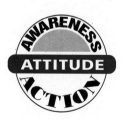

People

Emergency service is a people business. You have no choice about the people you deal with. They may be sick or angry or afraid, drunk or violent. They can be demanding, ungrateful, even abusive. You often encounter people at their worst.

It isn't just dealings with the public that causes stress. You have to get along with those in your department or squad, frequently under trying circumstances. Conflict is inevitable. Stress is the result.

Awareness—

What are the most common sources of conflict?

Attitude—

"I have my personal space where I feel comfortable. I act toward people from a position of strength and respect."

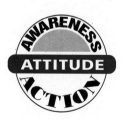

Action—

Communicate. Talk to people and tell them how you feel. If they're getting on your nerves, tell them so directly. At the same time, listen to what they're telling you.

Home Life

Your home should be a safe haven, a place to kick back and let go of the day's stress. Is it?

Relationships are difficult. Children are demanding. Marriages inevitably travel sections of rough road. Maybe there's a conflict between your home life and your emergency work.

Suddenly the place where you should be getting rid of your stress becomes a source of additional conflict and tension. **When was the last time you sat down with your spouse, or someone close to you, and talked about "us?"**

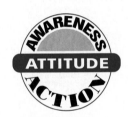

Awareness—

Do I feel safe and comfortable at home?

Attitude—

"I can put my worries aside when I go home. I'm determined to make it a place where I can relax and be myself."

Action—

Create a space at home that's exclusively yours: a den, a study, a workshop.

Burnout

A nurse who came for counseling put it this way: "It wasn't any one thing that bothered me. It was everything: work, money, time pressure. You name it, I had it. Then on the ambulance one night, this young kid died on me while I was holding his hand.

"Now I feel like my batteries are dead. I have no energy, no desire. I just don't care anymore."

A switchboard can handle only so many calls at one time. If more calls come in, the circuits will overload. Malfunctions will occur.

Cumulative stress is the enemy of emergency responders. You can cope with stress for a period of time. But sooner or later, if you do nothing about it, you reach a point of overload. It may take months. It often takes years.

A sump pump will keep a cellar dry as long as the flow of water is not faster than the pump's capacity. If water comes in faster than the pump can get rid of it, the result is overload—and a wet basement.

When stress comes at you from too many sources at once, it can get ahead of your coping mechanism. You don't adjust fast enough, stress builds up, you become overloaded.

You can be overloaded with stress and still function. But you're like a rocket with a limited amount of fuel. When the fuel burns out, the rocket slows down. Gravity then pulls it back to earth.

Burnout, the emotional exhaustion that results from overload, is a very real and constant danger for emergency responders. It can affect your job performance, turn you cynical and unproductive, take you out of service. It can have an even more serious impact on other areas your life, play havoc with your emotions, poison your relationships, demolish your self-image.

Burnout attacks your body, too. Heart disease. Ulcers. Migraines. Stress has even been implicated in some forms of cancer. Stress can, quite literally, kill you.

> *cumulative stress* Stress resulting from numerous stress reactions, which build up faster than your system can cope with them.

Fast Burn or Slow Burn?

Burnout sometimes happens all at once. The massive attack of stress from a single critical incident overwhelms your defenses. For example, a young woman who had been on a volunteer rescue squad for only five months was called to the scene of a grisly multi-casualty incident. She wasn't prepared for the horror and death she faced. She was overwhelmed and needed immediate crisis intervention.

More often, your circuits overload gradually. Stress accumulates from many directions, many areas of your life. At first you have no problem keeping all the balls in the air. But a point comes when there are just too many balls.

A single event may push you over the edge, bring the burnout home to you. It could be a particularly bad call, a death. It could be a series of bad calls. It could be something as simple as an argument with a colleague.

It's important to note that the straw that breaks the camel's back is not the real problem. A camel can certainly support a straw. The problem is, the camel is already overloaded. It's not the straw but the load that does the damage.

A man who is an electrical design engineer and volunteer fire captain told this story:

"I was senior design engineer on a major project due Jan. 15. This project was crucial to the survival of my company. From early fall my boss had questioned me daily about the status of the project. Each time, he reminded me of its importance. The stakes were high: my co-workers, even their families would be affected.

"On Dec. 23, I was completing my Christmas shopping at the mall. I'd been busy all week. The deadline was looming. Also, during the week my fire company had responded to a working house fire at two in the morning. Two of my men were injured at the scene and had to be hospitalized. I needed to get the insurance and compensation reports out.

"I left the store at 10 p.m. It was cold. A light snow was falling. I saw that the left rear of my car was sitting low. I walked around. Sure enough. Flat tire. I tossed the packages inside. I couldn't have cared less if something broke.

"I opened the trunk. What do you think? The spare was flat, too. I'd had it. I slammed the trunk shut. I walked over and crashed my hand into the rear window."

Welcome to the world of burnout. This man fractured his right hand and wrist. Because he was right-handed, the injury prevented him from contributing to the completion of the crucial project.

burnout The signs and symptoms of cumulative stress that begin to appear when the individual can no longer cope.

Was it the flat spare tire that the man was reacting to? No. That was the straw. He was a victim of cumulative stress. Overload took him to the breaking point. A single incident pushed him over the edge.

Awareness—

- What's important in my life?
- How can I manage things so that I can concentrate on my priorities and not feel pressured?

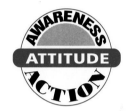

Attitude—

"I'm handling all the things I have to take care of as best I can. I can only do one thing at a time. I have to flow with whatever happens."

Action—

1. Prevent overload by relieving yourself of some pressure in advance. What's really important? This man could have done his holiday shopping by mail-order or assigned the department paperwork to his lieutenant.

2. Stress drove this man to a self-destructive act. When you feel that a minor incident is pushing you over the edge, always step back and take a few deep breaths. Venting your anger at this point will almost always increase your stress.

3. A good phrase to remember for these times is, "What's the worst that can happen?" For this man it was a minor expense, a wait for a tow truck, a late night. Hardly worth a broken wrist.

Stages of Burnout

Burnout does not always happen as suddenly and dramatically as it did with this man. Often it builds. You pass through different stages, with specific related symptoms.

It doesn't hit everyone the same way, but these four stages are common:

1. **The Honeymoon Stage.** You're gung-ho. You're enthusiastic. Emergency service gives you real pleasure. You're out on every call. When you return you pull the textbook out to see where you could have done better.

    You may even overdo it at this stage. You put so much energy into your emergency work that you neglect other areas of your life. You're planting the seeds of later problems.

2. **The Disillusionment Stage.** Your expectations begin to work against you. The people you help aren't always grateful. You can't always control the outcome of a situation. You encounter obstacles. You're forced to compromise.

    You're still out there, but you're a little more callous, a little more short-tempered. You don't look forward to that next meeting, that next training session.

3. **The Brown-Out Stage.** Your energy begins to flag. Your view of emergency service dims. The thought that enters your mind now is: *"Who cares?"* The routine bores you. Patients and colleagues annoy you. You don't crack the textbook anymore. Why should you?

    One EMT in this stage stated, *"I can't stand it when they whine."* He was referring to the victims of accidents. His compassion had dried up. In fact, everybody around him seemed to be whining lately.

4. **Total Burnout.** *"I think this guy planned his heart attack just to drag me out on a rainy night,"* a paramedic said. This is the stage of total frustration. Nobody can do anything right. You are actively hostile to those who seek your help—they're just objects to you. You have no energy at all. Everything requires an effort. You do only enough to get by. You become slack in your procedures. You don't care.

You've probably seen these stages in others. Take a close look at yourself. Are you headed toward burnout? Which stage are you in? Begin to think about taking some positive steps to keep from moving down that road.

You can help the new members in your squad or department keep off this downward slope toward burnout. Let them know that their expectations may be unrealistic, that what happens in the field is not the same as what's described in the textbook. Help prepare them for the powerful feelings that emergency work can generate. Help them to talk about their feelings.

Is Burnout a Defense?

In a way it is. A stress reaction is a form of compensation. You've learned about physical shock: the body closes down systems and organs in order to preserve circulation to the brain. In the case of burnout, your mind compensates for overload by closing down your capacity to care. You lose empathy with the patients you treat or the people you help. You isolate to avoid the pain.

But going into shock does not cure a person of his underlying problem. Shock is an indicator of big trouble. It's a desperate attempt to keep the body alive. It's time for anti-shock trousers, IV's, lights and siren.

In the same way, burnout, and the cynical attitude that goes along with it, is no cure. It's a sign that something is out of balance in your life. It's a sign that the tools you are using to cope with stress are inadequate.

The Importance

An EMS worker walks a tightrope. You need a certain distance from your patients, an objectivity. If you were to become personally involved with every person you care for, you would quickly deplete your emotional reserves. At the same time, to take the attitude, "I have to be callous to cope," can be equally dangerous. It prevents you from expressing, or even acknowledging to yourself, the real and quite normal reactions you have toward what you're doing.

The balancing pole that you carry on this tightrope is your professionalism. A professional attitude allows you to treat each patient with warmth and compassion. When you've given that patient the best treatment you can, you are able to step back, detach yourself emotionally, and continue with your life.

This professionalism comes with experience. But it's important for you to maintain your awareness. How do you view your patients? Are you too involved? Have you assumed an impenetrable armor against all sympathy with them? Are you too quick to resort to cynical humor in order to deny your feelings?

# of Professionalism

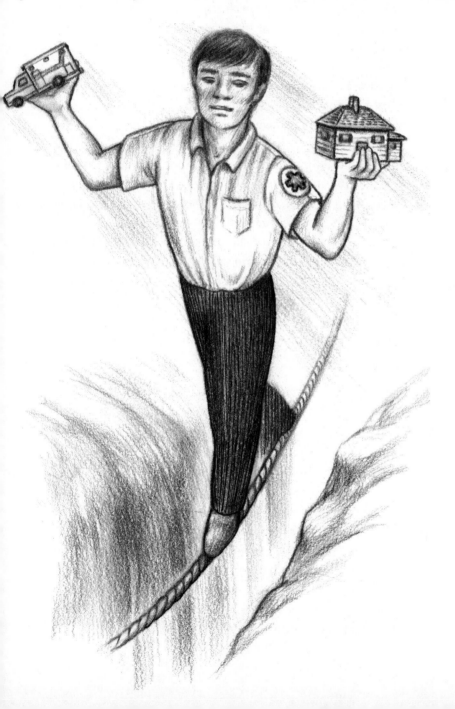

Burnout Takes Over

Burnout would be bad enough if it was confined to the emergency service area of your life. But just as the stress originates from many separate sources, stress can affect all of the facets of your life as well.

The wife of a paramedic stated:

"I don't know him anymore. He isn't the man I married five years ago. I married him because he was a loving, kind person. He always seemed to care about me and the children.

"Now he thinks only of himself. He spends hours in front of the TV. He's distant from all of us, never has a kind word for anyone.

"Last week our 4-year-old daughter fell off her bike in front of the house. We heard the screams. He looked up from the TV and made no attempt to see what had happened.

"When I got to her I could see that her wrist looked broken. I screamed for my husband. He slowly emerged from the front door, loomed over our daughter, and shouted, "Stop crying!" I can still see the look on his face.

"At that moment I realized he was someone I didn't know. Our daughter broke her hand and wrist in the fall. I think the stranger she calls Daddy broke her heart."

Stress is insidious. You start by being short with patients, with those who call for help. You end up where this man did, bringing the effects of stress home with you, letting burnout take over your life.

Your social life suffers. You no longer feel attached to your friends. One police officer in the latter stages of burnout found himself checking automobile inspection stickers on his way into a party he'd been invited to. "No slack," he said. "Anybody I see, if they're in violation, I write them a ticket." When this same officer came in for counseling, he made a revealing statement. "Nothing seems right anymore. I can't stand my job. I fight with my wife and kids. I don't like me much either."

I don't like me.

In the end, burnout tears down your self-image. You don't like who you are. You lose your sense of worth.

It's easy to see the snowball effect of stress. When burnout prompts you to write tickets on your friends when you're not on duty, you aren't going to be the most popular guy on the block. The result? Conflict and isolation. These produce further stress, adding to your already overloaded system. Meanwhile, low energy and low self-esteem block you from taking effective actions against your stress.

We're talking about something very powerful here.

Awareness—

When burnout reaches its advanced stages, it's very hard for you to kick it, or even recognize it, on your own. The first step is to talk it over with someone—a friend, a co-worker, someone you trust. Tell them what's been happening, how you feel. Ask them, "How am I doing?"

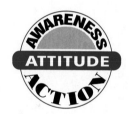

Attitude—

"I'm going to be good to myself and pull back before I reach the point of complete burnout. It makes sense not to push myself over the edge."

Action—

1. Sometimes at this point it's crucial for you to temporarily step away from your emergency service work. Take a leave of absence, a short vacation. Better to take time off than to reach the point where you abandon EMS work completely.

2. To prevent burnout from going this far, look for the signs. You can become burned out without necessarily feeling highly stressed. Survey yourself regularly for evidence that you're being overwhelmed.

The Alarm Bells

Stress can produce a wide variety of symptoms. They range from absent-mindedness to chest pains, from outbursts of anger to crying spells.

You know from your EMS work that physical conditions have both signs—things you can observe—and symptoms—things the patient feels. Pain is a symptom. Flushed skin is a sign. Stress often has symptoms. You feel "stressed out"—nervous, pressured, edgy.

But many of the indicators of stress are signs. You're drinking more alcohol than usual. You find yourself arguing with your spouse. You don't feel tense, but have frequent stomach pains. It's not always easy to recognize stress when it hits you.

> **Stress is an unavoidable part of life. It's natural, inevitable, and to be expected by all of us.**

Everyone who has responded to calls involving possible heart attack victims knows that the patient often denies that he or she is having an attack. Denial is common with stress as well. Many people, emergency responders in particular, are reluctant to admit that they "can't handle it." They feel that to acknowledge that stress is getting the best of them means to confess to weakness.

Awareness is crucial. You need to be on the lookout for signs of stress in yourself and in the people you work with. These are the six most common indicators in cases of burnout. They should serve as your alarm bells:

Sleep disturbances. You can't sleep. When you do get to sleep, you wake up frequently. Vivid, disturbing dreams jar you. You suffer from the "3 a.m. heebie-jeebies," black thoughts that pursue you as you lie awake.

Withdrawal. You turn away from co-workers, friends, family members. You'd rather be by yourself. You don't contribute anything at meetings. You don't participate in the activities you used to enjoy.

Fatigue. A paramedic reported that he would come off duty, eat dinner, hit his easy chair, and not move until it was time to go to bed. He was sleeping more than he ever had, but he was always tired.

Apathy. You just don't care anymore. You stop trying to improve your skills. You neglect your appearance. You are unmoved by what happens around you. Someone dies in your ambulance, it's just another call. Your department receives an award, you get no pleasure from it.

Physical symptoms. Remember that while physical symptoms may be caused by stress, they are very real. Don't dismiss chest pains as "just stress." See your doctor first, then start dealing with your stress.

Changes. The person who used to be talkative turns quiet. The EMT who was always first on the scene is now usually last. The paramedic who was a stickler for procedures becomes sloppy taking vital signs. The police officer who used to have an occasional beer after work now drinks a six-pack every night. Changes—in personality, behavior, mood—are a key alarm sign of burnout. Look for them in yourself and in your colleagues.

Stress Indicators: A Checklist

Below are some of the signs and symptoms that may indicate that you are being affected by stress. Use this checklist to conduct a stress assessment. Go through it periodically in order to record changes. Remember that none of these indicators by themselves point to overload or burnout. You're looking for a pattern.

☑ Behavior

Heavy smoking	Nightmares
Increased use of alcohol	Overwork
Drug use	Conflict with spouse
High-risk behavior	Outburst of anger
Violence	Crying spells
Overeating	Withdrawal from friends
Hyperactivity	Abrupt changes
Sleep disturbances	Startle reaction

☑ Attitude

Boredom	Critical toward self, others
Grandiosity	
Cynicism	Sarcasm
Distrust	Failing to see deeper meaning
Despair	
Feelings of powerlessness	Giving up on values
	Feeling trapped
Self-righteousness	Self-doubt

☑ Emotion

Anxiety

Feeling of being
  overwhelmed

Fear, paranoia

Feeling out of control

Guilt

Depression

Anger

Panic

Feeling disconnected
  from emotions

Feelings of tension,
  pressure

☑ Physical

Headaches

Stomach problems

Indigestion

Diarrhea

Nausea

Fatigue

Frequent colds

Weight loss or gain

Muscular pains

Changes in menstrual cycle

Shaking

Sweating

Heart palpitations

Vision problem

☑ Mental

Difficulty concentrating

Distractibility

Inability to make
  decisions

Short attention span

Intrusive images

Hyper-alertness

Self-blaming

Distorted thinking

Frequent daydreams

Avoidance of certain
  thoughts

☑ Other signs

Over dependence on
  others

Marital/relationship
  problems

Restricted social contacts

Lowered sex drive

Awareness—

Just as patient assessment is the most important skill of an EMT, recognition of overload and burnout is crucial to your efforts to cope and stay in service. Approach it systematically. Go through the warning signs and take a careful look at your life.

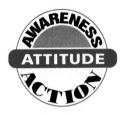

Attitude—

"Stress can get the better of me before I know it if I'm not on the lookout for the warning signs. I need to be vigilant."

Action—

1. Compare your current condition to the way you were in the past. What's changed? Why?
2. Occasionally ask your spouse or someone close to you to evaluate you for signs of stress. Sometimes others will see the changes before you do.

Now the Good News

Is burnout the fate of every emergency responder? Here's the account of a 23-year veteran firefighter:

"I love my job. I've loved it since the first day I arrived. It's tough at times, sometimes depressing, often rewarding. I never have a dull day. I have vowed to have a good life. I realize that I have to make it count this trip, because there is no second chance.

"The thing I believe has worked best for me is to make sure I have time for myself and for my family. When I leave the station at the end of my tour, I try to leave the job there. Sometimes, when we have a really dirty call, that isn't possible. On those days, I allow myself some extra time to unwind. I make an entry in my journal. I go for a walk.

"My hobby is sailing during the summer, skiing in the winter. Days off you will find me and my wife on the boat, down at the ocean. In winter, we ski as often as time and funds allow.

"My wife and I have a good relationship. We are able to talk about many things, including work. She is my support system when my feelings are low. We laugh. We have fun. I think this offsets much of the negative things I see at work.

"Burnout? I don't think so. I've worked hard at keeping a balance in my life."

Balance. Think about it. Stress comes from all areas of your life. Burnout can affect all areas of your life. The solution is to evaluate and bring into balance all areas of your life.

You are a total person. Emergency service is only one part of you. The key to coping with stress, to preventing burnout, is balance.

This firefighter balances work and fun. He balances his professional and his home life. He balances what he gives to his community and what he gives to himself.

The result? Instead of surrendering to disillusionment and apathy, he's been able to maintain his enthusiasm and stay in service for more than two decades.

The key to coping with stress, to preventing burnout, is balance.

SUMMARY

- The traits that make you a good emergency responder can also contribute to stress.
- Sometimes it takes strength to give up control.
- Your expectations have to be tempered with realism.
- Talking about the images you encounter in your emergency work helps defuse them as sources of stress.
- Cumulative stress can result in overload and burnout.
- Sources of stress include your "boss," deadlines, your job, money worries, people and domestic problems.
- Burnout may happen quickly, but usually occurs in stages.
- Balance is the key to dealing with emergency service stress.
- It's important to be aware of the symptoms of stress, especially the alarm bells:

  Sleep disturbances   Apathy

  Withdrawal   Physical symptoms

  Fatigue   Changes

For Further Thought ———————

1. Most of us know people who have dropped out of emergency service because it just became too much of a burden. Can you identify traits in those persons that might have contributed to their stress? How could they have handled it differently?

2. What are some reasons people are afraid to express their genuine feelings?

3. What are some specific sources of stress in your EMS job? Your relationships? Your life in general? How can a combination of Awareness, Attitude and Action keep each one from overwhelming you?

4. What are some ways to balance a genuine concern for patients with an ability to avoid becoming emotionally involved with every case?

5. Cite specific instances in which the six alarm bells of stress might show up in your life or that of your co-workers.

6. The fight or flight reaction is automatic, but may not be appropriate. Describe some scenarios when this is the case.

7. What are some disappointments that every EMS worker will face during his or her career?

CHAPTER 4

The Five Realms of the Total Person

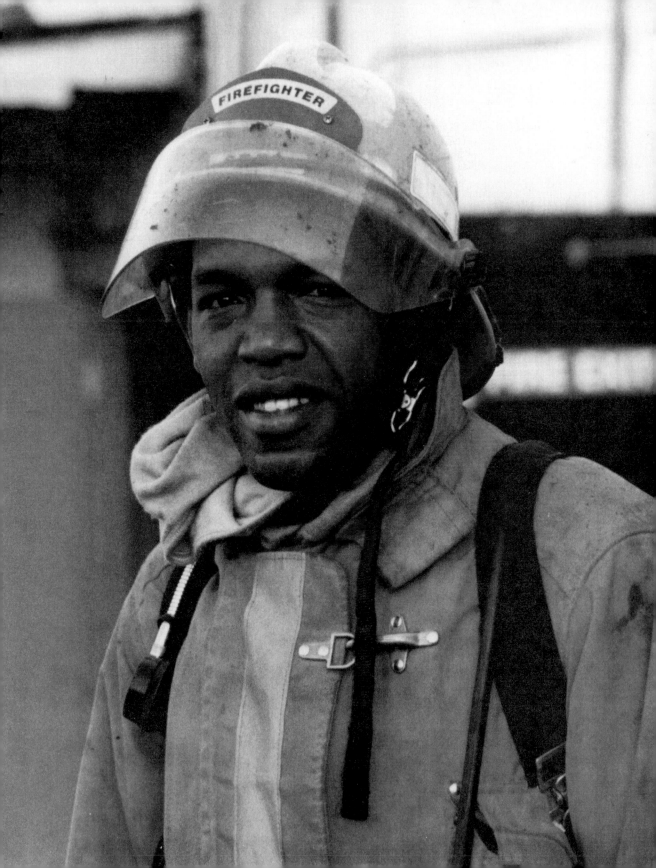

The Five Realms of the Total Person

Before you ever thought of entering emergency service, you were a total person, with the needs, worries, hopes, and problems that are shared by everyone walking the planet. You have been that person since you were born.

What does it take to stay in service? Training, you might say. Of course. Drills. The right equipment. Communications. Maintenance.

All of these elements are needed to serve others in emergencies. But there's an even more crucial component: **Yourself.** You have to be fit in both body and mind. You have to maintain yourself. You have to prepare yourself to deal with the stressful situations you will encounter on and off the job.

MENTAL

EMOTIONAL

PHYSICAL

SOCIAL

SPIRITUAL

A Question of Balance

A human being is a complicated creature. We all have five basic realms in our lives: the **social, emotional, mental, physical and spiritual.**

These are not separate entities within us. Rather, they are integrated facets of the **Total Person**. Each area is affecting all the other areas all the time.

total person The idea that the various components of your life are interconnected.

Imagine that you have a wound in your right leg. Is that the only part of your body affected? No. The pain distracts you. You can't concentrate. You grow irritable. If the wound becomes infected, you develop a fever throughout your body. You are one organism. An injury has an impact on your entire system.

This is true of stress as well. Stress can touch any of the five areas of your Total Person. The result is to throw you out of balance. All the other areas of your life may be affected.

Many emergency service people tend to divide their lives into compartments. They imagine that a conflict during a call has nothing to do with an argument they might have with their spouse the next night. They respond to a fatal accident, then wonder why a week later while watching television tears suddenly spring to their eyes

Think of a car. The front end is out of alignment. The problem doesn't stop there. Steering becomes difficult. The tires wear unevenly. If nothing is done, a blow-out may throw the car out of control.

You might identify with the story told by an EMT who was suffering from stress:

"I have a wife, two children, a house with high monthly payments, and a bunch of other bills coming in. I want my family to have it good, so I work as hard as I can to make the payments, keep things going.

"I thought I had to work as many hours as I could. That way we could get ahead of the bills, have some of the extra things.

"Looking back, I see that in the process of working extra hard I almost lost my family. My wife and I became strangers. I barely had time to be with my children. I became depressed, irritable, distant."

This person learned that balance is a crucial part of withstanding stress. His motives were good, but by putting so much energy into one area of his life—earning a living—he neglected another crucial aspect, his relationship with his family.

Balance is an antidote to stress. The key is to regularly pay attention to the five facets of your life. Keep an eye on how you're coping. Correct problems in each area as they arise.

The Domino Effect

You're worried about money, so you overwork. Because you overwork, you're always tired. You make mistakes. You become irritable. Your irritation creates conflicts with your co-workers. These conflicts make you angry. Others avoid you, you become isolated. Fatigue wears down your immune system. You develop the flu.

Each domino knocks down another. A single source of stress has an impact on many facets of your life.

This is a crucial fact to keep in mind: Stress spills over. The only way to keep stress from toppling your dominos is to work at maintaining balance in all the areas of your Total Person.

"Nothing is Right"

Mary was 30 years old. She was trained as a nurse, worked on an ambulance as a paramedic. She came for counseling because stress had knocked over all her dominos. The imbalance in her life had overwhelmed her.

Eight years earlier, her husband Jim had left for work one morning. He kissed her and the kids goodbye the way he always did. 'I'll see you later,' he said.

Later never came. A drunk driver hit Jim head-on. He was killed instantly. At 22, Mary was a widow with two young children.

"In a heartbeat my entire world caved in," she said.

Her family and friends supported her. She pulled her life together. The wound seemed to heal. But Mary never fully resolved the grief she felt over Jim's death. The incident left her with the seeds of stress that would bear fruit years later.

After hearing a presentation of the Total Person concept, Mary stated, "*I thought you were talking about me. I'm about as far out of balance as you can get.*"

This was the story she told:

"*About two years ago I met John. I had not allowed myself to date for a very long time after Jim died. He had been the first and most important man in my life. I couldn't begin to think of allowing someone to take his place.*

"*But the time came when I was ready to date again. John entered my life. He was a great guy. My kids liked him, he liked them. Everything seemed to be on track. For the first time since Jim's death I allowed myself to become emotionally involved. I began to think about marrying John.*

"*Last month, John came over for dinner. I knew something wasn't right. He seemed on edge. After dinner, when the kids were in bed, he said, 'We need to talk.'*

"*My heart sank. I knew something was coming. He told me he'd gotten the promotion he'd been waiting for. He was being transferred to California.*

"*For a minute, I was delighted. I thought that moving to California would be great. But in the next breath he said it: 'I'm sorry—you won't be coming with me.'*

"*I felt a knife plunge into my gut. I was angry. I was shocked. I didn't believe what I'd heard. How could this be happening to me again? It had taken me so long to commit to a relationship. When I finally did—it collapsed.*"

The Social Realm

Mary's problems began when stress overwhelmed the social area of her Total Person. The immediate cause was the breakdown of her relationship with John. The deeper source was the unresolved grief she felt over Jim. The social difficulties faced by any single mother also contributed.

Relationships are demanding, complicated, sometimes frustrating. Other people are not always dependable. Each of us faces the constant challenge of forming and maintaining connections to others, of getting along with people. This can be a potent source of stress.

Emergency service adds to stress in the social realm. It brings us into contact with people who are themselves under stress. We see people at their worst. The nature of the work makes demands on our relationships with family members and friends. It can come between spouses. It can keep parents from spending enough time with their children.

Each of us faces the constant challenge of forming and maintaining connections to others.

Isolation is easy. Relationships, as Mary found, are hard and unpredictable.

The Emotional Realm

Mary's problems didn't stay contained within the social area of her life. Her emotional realm was thrown out of balance. She displayed anger. She would become suddenly depressed. She cried a lot. She was on an emotional roller coaster.

This was her second domino. Her emotional disturbance fed back to increase the stress in her social realm. She would scream at her children. She became irritable with patients, she fought with co-workers.

EMS often throws you into highly charged emotional situations.

Emergency service makes demands on the emotional facet of the Total Person. It often throws you into highly charged emotional situations. But you are expected to maintain rigorous self-control. You see and experience events that set off powerful emotional reactions within you.

Finding an outlet for these feelings is not always easy. That's why the emotional realm is easily thrown out of balance by stress.

The Mental Realm

Mary would get into her car and go to the store. When she arrived, she couldn't remember the drive there. Her mind was a blank. She couldn't even remember why she'd come. *"I'm in a fog that won't lift,"* she said.

Even worse, she began to administer the wrong medications to her patients. Once she had to apply a traction splint and couldn't remember the steps. She couldn't make decisions—about what to wear, what to eat, what to do.

Unresolved stress quickly affects your ability to concentrate. You become like that switchboard with the overloaded circuit—nothing gets through. You make simple mistakes. You are plagued by repetitive thoughts.

> *Unresolved stress quickly affects your ability to concentrate.*

Emergency service amplifies stress in the mental realm. You have to remember a host of procedures and other information. You are frequently faced with life-or-death decisions. You must concentrate in the midst of chaos. Often you have to improvise, think on your feet when time is pressing.

Mental stress spills over. You stand up to speak before a group and your mind goes blank. The pressure to remember so many facts for a state EMT certification test comes out in anxiety, irritability, maybe even physical illness. The worries and second thoughts that come after a complicated call can keep you up at night.

The Physical Realm

This is the most frightening part of Mary's story. She did not look well. She was gaunt, pasty, tremulous. She'd lost 32 pounds in six weeks.

"I can't eat," she said. *"If I do, 10 minutes later I'm in the bathroom losing whatever I did eat. After giving up smoking for six years, I'm back to two packs a day. I haven't slept a solid five hours since John walked out."*

Another domino. Mary's social stress had hit her physical realm. The connection between stress and physical health is now well established. It may show up as something severe—heart problems or ulcers. It may result in digestive difficulties. It may cause aches and pains, a tendency to have frequent colds.

Emergency service puts many physical demands on you. Just jumping out of bed and rushing to a fire or motor vehicle accident at three o'clock on a winter morning is physically stressful. You are called on to drag hose, to lift patients, to carry Indian packs into brush fires, to operate for hours at the scene of a disaster.

Everyone knows how hard it is to ignore a toothache or a backache. Just as stress creates physical symptoms, physical problems can ripple through your Total Person, setting off stress in many areas.

> *The connection between stress and physical health is well established.*

The Spiritual Realm

Mary had been raised with a deep belief in God. She was an active member of her church. She taught Sunday school. She took her kids to church and prayed with them at home. Since John left, she'd stopped attending church.

"How could there be a God?" she asked. *"A loving God would not have done this to me twice in my life. I did all the things God wanted. It's all a bunch of junk."*

She felt a conflict between her spiritual anger and her deeper faith. This conflict further complicated her emotional and mental distress.

The spiritual realm includes more than religion. This is the area of your life in which you deal with the meaning of things. It has to do with the mysteries of life —birth, death, love, fate—the areas where reason and science can't provide all the answers.

> *The spiritual realm is the area of your life in which you deal with the meaning of things.*

In emergency service you have many profound experiences. You come into contact with courage, heroism, acts of deep compassion. You also see people die. You see illness and despair. You see how carelessness or a whim of fate can snuff out a life.

These experiences can affect your spiritual beliefs. They can make you ask difficult and complicated questions about life and what it means. Again, you need to find a balance. This is not an area you can neglect.

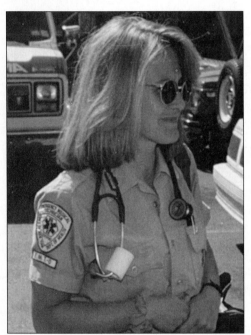

Tending to the Total Person

Keep in mind that stress comes in many varieties. Some of the stess you will experience will be of a "garden variety." This is the result of events that occur in your ordinary daily life, like traffic jams, schedule conflicts, or a flat tire. These things might build up or aggravate, but not fundamentally change you. They can be handled easily if you apply your coping skills.

Major life events are a far more serious source of stress. The death of a loved one, a serious illness or injury, the loss of a job, or a very serious incident that you respond to in your EMS work—these will tax to the limit your powers to cope.

The stress of major life events—the kind of stress that Mary faced—can quickly spill over from one realm of your life into all the others. For Mary, stress in the social realm eventually affected every facet of her life.

To cope with stress and its effects you need to pay attention to each area. Don't just focus on the symptoms. Look for the underlying cause. Look at the way the stress is affecting each part of you.

To be healthy, the Total Person—the person behind the uniform—requires harmony in all areas. This harmony, this balance is the best antidote for stress.

Consider the case of a police officer who sought counseling. His problem? He would break into tears at inappropriate times.

"I hear a song on the radio and suddenly I can't stop bawling," he said. His emotional realm was out of whack. But as he talked about himself, other facts came out:

"My father died from heart disease when he was 47. My uncle suffered a coronary at 49. My grandfather dropped dead at 42. My grandmother died when she was 44.

"Know how old I am? Forty-one. Two weeks ago, when I was walking up a flight of stairs, I felt a sharp pain in the middle of my chest. I know what angina is. I'm afraid to go to the doctor about it."

The source of his stress was physical. He was worried about his heart—with good reason. That stress spilled over. It left him an emotional wreck. It affected his ability to concentrate on his job. It threw him out of balance.

Your task is to survey your Total Person at regular intervals. Turn to each realm of your life and ask the question: **How am I doing?**

Physical

Sometimes problems will show up in the form of acute symptoms, such as angina or migraines. Often, the physical signs of stress consist of minor indications—fatigue, frequent colds, poor digestion.

Awareness—

- How is my general health? Has it changed for the worse?
- How am I sleeping?
- Do I suffer from frequent insomnia?
- Do I feel refreshed in the morning?
- Does my jaw ache from clenching my teeth all night?
- Do I fall asleep on duty?
- Am I bothered by diarrhea? Nausea? Indigestion?
- Do I take the time to eat my meals slowly?

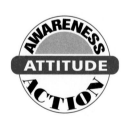

- Do I get enough exercise? Am I fit enough to meet the demands of my job?
- Do I accept my physical limits? Or do I strain myself by overdoing it?

Attitude—

"I can take responsibility for many areas of my health. Healthy habits pay immediate benefits. Long-term they play a big role in helping me cope with stress."

Action—

1. Get out and walk every day. This is the single most effective way to restore physical balance.
2. Cut out greasy and sugar-laden foods.
3. Limit your alcohol intake to one or two drinks a day.
4. If you smoke, see how long you can go each day before lighting up.
5. Go easy on the coffee and soda.
6. Begin a program of regular swimming—one of the best forms of exercise.
7. Visit your doctor for a full physical to dispel nagging health worries.
8. Take an "oxygen break." Step back from what you're doing and spend a minute taking deep, full breaths.

Emotional

An interesting way to evaluate your emotional health is to imagine that a video camera has been installed in every room in your house. Surveillance is also being conducted on the job—in your ambulance, fire station, or patrol car. What kind of person would a day's tape show? Someone who is generally happy and amiable? Or a short-tempered, depressed cynic?

Awareness—

- Am I happy? A simple question but a key one.
- Do I react in most cases with the appropriate emotion?
- Do I have a short fuse? Do I periodically explode with anger?
- Do I sometimes cry for no real reason?
- When was the last time I expressed my real feelings?
- Am I frequently depressed?
- Do my moods vary wildly?

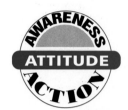

Attitude—

"Holding in emotions is not necessarily a sign of strength. I am sometimes strong enough to let go and express my feelings."

Action—

1. A couple of times every day, step back and examine how you feel.
2. Set aside some time to be good to yourself—to do the things you enjoy.
3. Look at your values: What's important to you? Are your priorities in line with your values?
4. Keep a journal of your emotional status. Note when you feel "off," when you are containing feelings.
5. Touch people more—physically and emotionally. A hand on an arm, a hug, a shared joke or disappointment.
6. Set aside a few minutes every day to be alone. Learn to benefit from solitude.
7. Develop a source of enthusiasm: get out to see a local sports team or coach Little League. Cheering is an excellent way to release emotional energy.

Mental

Your mind works best when it acts as a spotlight, focusing on one thing at a time. Stress interferes with your ability to concentrate. Take some time to listen to your inner monologue—the "voice" that keeps running through your head. Is it clear and coherent? Or is it cluttered, confused, full of static?

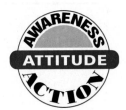

Awareness—

- Do I frequently "wake up" to find time has passed while I've been daydreaming?
- Am I forgetful? Do I often lose my keys, miss appointments?
- Do I have trouble making decisions?
- Am I focused on what occupies me at the moment?
- Am I bothered by obsessive or repetitive thoughts?
- Do I frequently become distracted or preoccupied?

Attitude—

"I can shut out the noise and distraction and focus on what I need to think about."

Action—

1. Take up a hobby unrelated to emergency work, anything from fishing to wood carving to gardening.
2. Become an "expert" on some subject—local history, Civil War battles, astronomy. Pick a field that allows you ample room to continue learning.
3. Find out about auditing courses at a local college.
4. Research your family's genealogy.

5. Learn a language.

6. Attend lectures offered at local museums or cultural institutes.

7. Take a "mental health day." Devote an entire day to getting a total break from your usual routine.

Social

A strong support system of close friends and family members can be one of the best defenses against stress. But too often, stress isolates us. As an emergency responder, you must be particularly careful not to allow your work to come between you and the people in your life who are important to you.

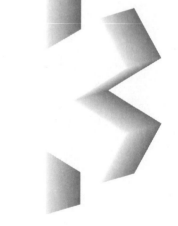

"Social Supports" is the term social scientists use to describe positive interaction among people. These exchanges may include passing along information, offering material support, or providing emotional support.

The health implications of these exchanges are especially important during periods of stress, life transitions, and crisis. More and more evidence demonstrates that peoples' relationships with their spouses, friends, families, colleagues, co-workers, and neighbors can buffer stress and have a positive effect on physical and mental health.

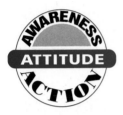

Awareness—

- Is there someone I could call right now and really talk with about the things that are bothering me?
- Is my social life completely tied to my emergency work?
- Do I trust other people?
- Do I share my problems with my spouse or other family members?
- Do I have a meaningful relationship with the special person in my life?
- Am I really open with the people I care about?
- Do I have a tendency to isolate myself?
- Do I get along with co-workers?

Attitude—

"My social contacts depend mostly on what I do. If I reach out to people they will respond."

Action—

1. Join a club or association of people with whom you share interests.
2. Call up a relative that you haven't spoken to for some time.
3. Arrange to do something different with the people you see regularly—go to the movies with people from your rescue squad, share Sunday brunch with your colleagues from work.
4. Learn to listen. Good listeners don't just refrain from dominating a conversation, they pay attention and think about what the other person is saying.
5. Get in touch with an old friend whom you haven't seen in some time.
6. Be sure to spend time regularly with people you like, people who don't make emotional demands on you.

Spiritual

You can neglect your spiritual realm even though you go to church every week. The question is whether you take enough time to reflect on this area and to become comfortable with your own sense of the meaning of things.

Awareness—

- Do I ever sit down with someone to talk about what really matters?
- Do I sometimes feel that I am searching for meaning without finding it?
- Have events left me with nagging doubts about spiritual matters?
- Have my beliefs or spiritual habits changed suddenly? Why?

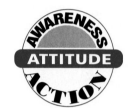

Attitude—

"My spiritual side needs and deserves the attention I give it."

Action—

1. Spend a few minutes every day reading scriptures or other books that are especially meaningful to you.
2. When you feel troubled, don't hesitate to talk to a member of the clergy or your agency's chaplain. That's what they're there for.
3. Consider a retreat, a period of time set aside for reflection.
4. Don't wait until Thanksgiving to give thanks. Make a list of the things that you have to be thankful for today.
5. Forgive yourself—it's just as important as forgiving others.
6. Buy a book that has meditations for each day. Tape a favorite thought to your bathroom mirror or over your desk.

Seeking Professional Help

Mary was smart. She realized that stress had spilled over to affect all facets of her life. She knew that she couldn't cope with the problems she faced in all these areas. She recognized the warning signs. She sought professional help.

III **Don't Be Afraid to Seek the Help of a Professional**

Working together with her therapist, Mary got a grip on the source of her distress. She learned to deal with its effects in the different realms of her Total Person. She began to move back toward health.

Emergency responders are the ones who are always urging people to call for help early. Don't make futile attempts to fight a structure fire. Dial 9-1-1. Don't ignore the warning signs of a heart attack. Call an ambulance. We offer this advice because we've seen the effects of waiting too long: the fully involved fire, the person in cardiac arrest.

So why do we ourselves delay or avoid calling on a professional to help with stress problems? It goes back to The Superhuman Myth. I can do it all.

Extreme symptoms in any of the five areas of your life can indicate stress problems that require outside help. For example, one firefighter was going through the pressure of a divorce and custody fight. He first began to feel "stressed out." He ignored it. Then he developed vision difficulties related to migraine headaches. He denied that he needed help. Later he was rushed to the hospital with an acute anxiety reaction and hyperventilation. Only then did he seek aid from a therapist.

Occasional anger or unhappiness should alert you to the need to put balance back into your life. But serious depression or rage bordering on violence mean you need help. Now.

Ask around. Friends, clergy, or your family doctor are the best sources of information about therapists in your area. Before you begin sessions with anyone, ask questions.

What is the person's background and experience? Does the therapist understand the special stress faced by emergency responders? How does the person plan to help you? How long will it take? How much will it cost? Will my insurance cover it?

There are two important points to remember when considering professional help for stress problems:

1. **Therapy is normal.** Seeking help does not mean you're crazy, nuts, or mentally ill. It means you've found the courage to address the difficulty you're experiencing. It's common sense to get advice from someone who has experience with the type of problems you're facing.

2. **What you get out is what you put in.** No therapist will magically cure you. The counseling relationship is a partnership in healing. It will take time. You'll need to work at the process.

Awareness—

- Do my problems seem overwhelming?
- Do I sometimes feel I'm never going to get my head above water again?
- What do my friends say? Are they giving me a message I don't want to hear?

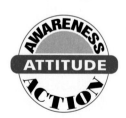

Attitude—

"Seeking professional help for stress or emotional problems is a sensible course of action. I don't need to feel embarrassed or weak."

Action—

Sometimes it's useful to determine in advance where you might go for help. Get together with some people in your squad and draw up a list of stress-counseling resources—therapists, psychologists, and other mental health professionals.

Wellness

We're used to looking at health and illness as opposites. It's black or white. It's either/or. Either I'm sick or I'm healthy.

The truth is that health is a continuum. At one end of the line is degenerative disease, imminent death. At the other end is optimum health and positive well-being. We all find ourselves somewhere along the line. The crucial question is: Where? And which way are we headed?

We call it health care. Many of us work in the health care system, jumping in to stabilize those patients who are slipping precariously close to the wrong end of the continuum.

What it should be called is sick care. The medical establishment is geared to returning patients from sick to neutral. Once a person is free of disease and can function, he's "cured." He may be overweight. He may smoke. He may be living a life marred by conflict and unhappiness. But he's classified as healthy.

The idea of wellness simply states that everyone can and should be moving toward optimum wellness. You should no more accept the neutral point as your goal than you should live with a curable disease.

wellness The idea that health is more than freedom from disease and that a person needs to take regular actions to increase physical and emotional well-being.

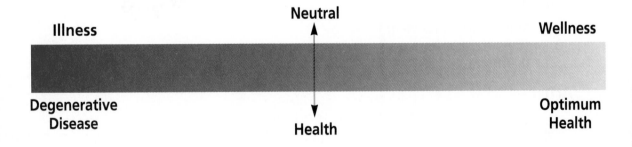

The Continuum of Wellness

Neutral

Illness   Wellness

Degenerative
Disease   Health   Optimum
                                                Health

Why Wellness?

Why should an emergency responder be interested in wellness? You've chosen an activity that tends to push you toward the illness end of the continuum. You're responding regularly to stressful events in your EMS work. You're spending long hours riding a patrol car in traffic. You're exposed to the strain and smoke of fighting serious fires. You need to take active measures to keep moving toward greater health.

You might even say that wellness is part of your job. One firefighter who keeps in good physical shape attended a debriefing following a major multi-casualty incident at a remote site. He had this to say to his fellow rescuers:

"You know, we joke about it all the time, the big gut hanging over our belts, the cigarette we drag on to clear our lungs after a smoky fire. The sad thing is, the guys with the bellies, the guys who smoke, they were the ones having some problems that night.

"I carried two five-gallon cans of gas a mile up a hill that night. I saw guys who had to sit down and rest just walking to the scene. One fireman had a heart attack climbing that hill.

"I know the toll this kind of thing takes on us. I don't claim to be in perfect condition. But I know one thing: If I had to, I could carry one of you out of a burning building."

If you aren't steadily moving toward wellness, the stress of emergency service is sooner or later going to catch up with you. Wellness does not eliminate stress from your life. It puts you in a better position to cope.

What is it that you're moving toward on the wellness end of the continuum?

- Freedom from disease and a resistance to illness.
- Greater ability to cope with stress from all sources.
- Positive feelings of contentment and happiness.

- A sense of accomplishment and growth.
- The awareness of a purpose to life.
- Self-respect and responsibility for your own health.

The idea of wellness is related to a saying: *"Enjoy life, this is not a dress rehearsal."* You are not practicing to live, the moments that make up your day are your life. And life is not an endurance contest, something just to get through. It should be savored. Wellness is an approach that lets you enjoy your life to the fullest.

Moving Toward Wellness

Wellness requires you to make an effort. If you do nothing you will never pass the neutral point on the continuum. There are four steps that lead you toward wellness. You must climb these steps not once but over and over if you are to achieve your goal of optimum health. This is the Staircase of Wellness.

Accept Change

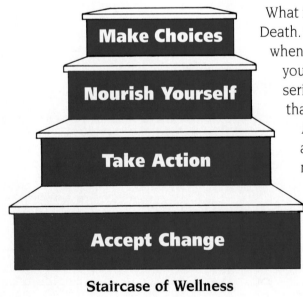

Make Choices

Nourish Yourself

Take Action

Accept Change

Staircase of Wellness

What in life is completely finished? The answer is: Death. Think about it. The process of life ends only when you die. Your stress will end only when you die. Until that point, your life is an endless series of changes. Change is the one thing that's guaranteed.

Accepting change as the substance of life is a crucial first step toward wellness. You are not static. You are not complete. You are not frozen in place by what has happened in the past. The single greatest obstacle to wellness is to look at yourself and to say, "I am this. I can't change." Your life is a process. Everything is a phase.

IV Don't Fight Change, Use it to Your Advantage

Accepting change opens vistas. Life becomes an opportunity for growth. You can try anything. A new job. New hobbies. Meet new people. Learn new things. Will you always succeed? No. Will there be pain and frustration? Of course. But there will be something else. Possibility. Hope.

One firefighter explained it this way:

"What sold me on the idea of change was simply to take a look at what we call the 'dinosaurs' in the department. Some of them are older guys, but not all. They like doing everything the way it's always been done. They resist new procedures. They don't like new equipment. They aren't open to new people. In the end they stagnate. The job has so little excitement for them. I don't want to be that way."

Accepting change keeps you from turning into a dinosaur. It helps you to see that next training session as an opportunity, not a chore. Maybe you have some ideas of your own to offer.

Change is important in maintaining the balance in your Total Person. Physical changes are inevitable. Are you maturing emotionally as well? Is your social life growing? Are you changing in terms of acquiring new knowledge and experience?

You only have two choices in life: change or stagnation. Your path to wellness begins when you accept change.

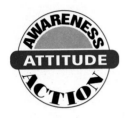

Awareness—

- How are you different than you were a year ago?
- What do you know now, about life and human nature, that you didn't know before?
- What changes do you face in the future?
- What opportunities might they present?

Attitude—

"Change is a part of life. Sometimes the change I will face will be welcome, and sometimes it will be difficult. I will effectively handle the change that comes my way."

Action—

Make a list of the changes that have happened to you recently. Think about how you handled each one.

Take Action

As an emergency responder you are action-oriented. So the second step toward wellness should come naturally to you. You have to do something. You have to turn change in a positive direction.

Again, this relates to your Total Person. When you identify an imbalance in one area of your life, you need to act to restore balance. The stress symptoms that we've already talked about are messages to you that you need to do something. They're calls to your body's 9-1-1 system.

For example, say you weigh a few pounds more than the ideal. You find yourself seriously short of breath walking upstairs. First, accept the fact that you are not permanently overweight, that you can change. Then take action: make changes in your diet, get on an exercise program, join a support group.

One professional paramedic told his partner he was thinking of giving up emergency work.

"It's my back," he said. *"It's gotten so bad I can't do the work any more. Forget about lifting patients, I can hardly carry the jump kit."*

"What have you done for it?" his partner asked.

"Nothing I can do. I just have a bad back. It's been that way for years. It's gotten worse and worse."

His partner did this person a favor. He gave him the name of an orthopedist. The doctor suggested a series of simple exercises. In six weeks the paramedic's back was noticeably better. He stayed in service. Action made the difference. By reading this book you are already taking action to deal with stress. Apply this "Can Do" attitude to all areas of your life. Identify where action is needed and do it.

Awareness—

- Are some of your stress problems the result of letting things slide?
- Do you spend more time worrying about problems than you do taking actions to remedy them?

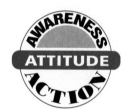

Attitude—

"Action is the best way to deal with stress. I'm not afraid of making mistakes. I tackle problems with confidence and a sense of purpose."

Action—

1. Take care of the unpleasant tasks first. Get them over with.

2. To stop procrastinating, use leading activities. Make a phone call, send for information, anything that gets you started on the project you've been avoiding.

3. Create your own deadlines.

4. Break projects into small parts and spend a little time with them every day.

Nourish Yourself

Your body needs food to live. If you're smart you eat a healthy diet. You take in enough of the various food groups to maintain balance in your system.

The day that you begin to take responsibility for your choices is the day you will take your biggest step toward wellness.

The rest of your Total Person needs nourishment, too. Actions are required to correct imbalances. Nourishment is needed to maintain balance. You don't wait until you're starving before you eat. A steady diet of nourishment for your mind and spirit is part of the climb toward wellness.

Nourish Your Mind As Well As Your Body

How do you nourish the various parts of your Total Person? First, don't neglect physical nourishment. The demands on you as an emergency responder are intense. You need to eat well, avoid excess fat and empty calories, in order to be ready to respond.

You nourish your mind by learning. Keep improving your emergency skills, sure. But go further. Take a course on some subject unrelated to your job. Read. Join an adult education program at your local college or school. Get involved in community affairs. Take up a new hobby.

The important point is to nourish all areas of your Total Person. Too often, the temptation is to focus on the emergency response aspect of your life—the meetings, drills, classes, social activities. This is like eating a diet that consists of only one food. It may fill you up, but it does not promote wellness.

Nourishment is preventive maintenance. When it comes to our equipment, we all understand the need for keeping it in top working order so that it doesn't fail us when we're at a fire or treating a patient. But when it comes to ourselves, we often take the attitude: If it ain't broke, don't fix it.

Wrong. To reach wellness, you need to maintain yourself, to nourish yourself before something goes wrong. It's only common sense.

Awareness—

- Look at what you are doing to nourish and maintain each area: social, emotional, mental, physical and spiritual.
- Is your diet out of balance?

Attitude—

"Prevention is better than cure. I don't wait for stress to overwhelm me in a particular area before I nourish that facet of my Total Person."

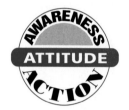

Action—

Make a list of activities that help maintain you in each facet of your life. Refer to it when you need nourishment in a given area.

Make Choices

"This job is making me crazy." Sound familiar?

"They made me do it." Maybe you've said it yourself.

"It's not me, it's them. It's the job. It's my boss. It's my family. It's life. I'm not responsible."

Everything you do in your life is a choice. You are the one who makes the choice. The day that you begin to take responsibility for your choices is the day you will take your biggest step toward wellness.

As an emergency responder, you've lived through situations in which someone's life was in your hands. It's time to realize that your own life is also in your hands.

Emergency service exposes you to stressful events—we all know that. Sometimes the events will be very powerful and will tax your coping mechanism to the limit. At other times it will not be those who have called you for help that cause the stress, it will be the choices and thoughts you are having about the situation.

As part of this step, you need to make the following statement part of your thinking:

> Neither he, she, they, or it
> makes me feel this way.
> The thoughts I am choosing
> make me feel this way.

Things will happen to you. Some of them will be unpleasant. You will experience loss. At times you will fail. You can't control that. What you can control is your response to what happens. Wellness means making choices.

"He made me so mad I flew off the handle." No. He did something you didn't like. You let your anger get out of control. You chose to fly off the handle.

Choice applies to every area of your Total Person. It's time to stop the blame game. No one is putting a gun to your head and forcing you to smoke, forcing you to eat a poor diet, or to flop on the couch instead of going for a walk. You choose what you do.

In the same way, no one is forcing you to bottle up your emotions. You choose not to express them. No one is forcing you to sit at home in front of the tube night after night. You are always making choices.

It's impossible to give up responsibility for your life. You are making choices all the time. Even if you do nothing, it's a choice. When you let an opportunity pass by, that's a choice. You can't avoid choices by sticking your head in the sand.

A woman who worked as a paramedic for 12 years told this story:

"I used to be one of these people with an attitude. I'd had a few set-backs in life, including a divorce. I thought the world was against me. Whether it was giving a little extra on the job or going back to school or whatever, I always had the idea: 'I can't do it.'

"One time we responded to a bad motor vehicle accident. The passengers were all teenagers. I treated a 15-year-old. She'd fractured one of her cervical vertebrae. She had no sensation in her lower extremities. We backboarded her and took her in.

"I didn't usually get involved with my patients, but I was concerned about this kid. I went to see her in the hospital later. She wasn't completely paralyzed but she'd lost a lot of movement in her legs. Lots of times when I stopped by she would be in the physiotherapy unit.

"I couldn't get over this kid's courage. Every step was painful for her, but she kept at it. The doctors doubted if she would ever walk again, but she kept trying. Some days she made a little progress, some days she seemed worse.

"Now, whenever I'm tempted to say 'I can't,' I imagine myself explaining to that girl why I can't. My excuses always seem pretty flimsy. Usually I end up telling myself, 'If I want to, I can.'"

Awareness—

- Do I constantly blame my problems on others?
- Do I often see bad luck or fate as responsible for the difficulties I encounter?
- Am I aware of the choices I make every day, even if they aren't conscious decisions?

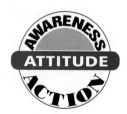

Attitude—

"I make choices every day and I take responsibility for them. I am the one who is in control of my life."

Action—

1. Make a list of the options that are open to you in a particular area of your life, such as your job or your social encounters. What are some choices you might make?

2. Then make a list of the obstacles and impediments to taking a particular course of action in that area. How can you take control of the situation by eliminating or bypassing the obstacles?

An Endless Process

Where does the Staircase of Wellness end? It doesn't. Once you've begun to make choices in your life, you'll realize that choices mean change. You've started all over again.

You can visualize it like walking up an escalator that's moving down. If you walk at the same pace the stairs are moving, you'll remain in one spot. If you walk faster, you'll move upward. But if you stop walking, you'll immediately slip back.

Life is change. Wellness is a process, a perpetual goal, not something you achieve through a one-time effort. Wellness is a way of living.

Maybe you've begun by realizing that you're in pretty sad shape physically. You accept the fact you can change. You take action by walking a mile every other day. You nourish yourself by eating right and cutting back on smoking. You say to yourself, *"Hey, I can do it. It's my choice."*

Now you realize you needn't stop there. You can keep making progress on the continuum. Maybe you join the YMCA and take up a swimming program. Maybe you start jogging a couple of miles a day. You make change happen. You get in better shape. Time passes and maybe you find yourself running in a 3-mile race. Even a marathon. Others have done it. You can. It's your choice.

Life is change. Wellness is a process, a perpetual goal, not something you achieve through a one-time effort. Wellness is a way of living.

Keeping Motivated

Some firefighters were sitting around talking about retirement. One man mentioned that he wasn't particularly looking forward to retirement. He was asked why.

"To me, retirement means you move to Florida and then you die."

The mind is a very powerful instrument. It affects your health. It affects the course of your life. If you believe something, it's likely that it will come true.

We all know people—maybe some quite close to us—for whom retirement did mark the end. They were never sick a single day when they were working. But now that they're retired you find them sick all the time. Maybe in a nursing home. Maybe sitting around the house with no purpose in life. Or maybe we visit them in the cemetery.

What happened? They came to the end. They lost purpose, stopped moving toward wellness, and slid back into illness.

Now consider a different story, this one told by an Advanced EMT:

"I met Sara when I was a junior in college. I knew there was something special about her. She would come to school every day by bus, an hour each way. She had a glow of life about her. She could talk to anyone on campus about any subject, from sports to world events. I'd rarely met a person who was so involved in life. The remarkable thing was: Sara was 80 years old.

"She'd returned to school after retiring from work at a local bank, a job she'd held for 42 years.

"'I always wanted to go to college,' she told me, 'but my parents didn't have the money. There were 12 kids in our family. I went to work at 17 to help the family get by. The years just sailed past. Now it's my turn. I've earned it.'

"She did earn it. She earned her bachelor's degree when she was 82. She went on to gain a master's at 85. And she was still coming to school by bus."

What's the difference between Sara and those who just give up and die? Motivation. Sara accepted the fact that life is change. She didn't say, "I'm too "old."

She knew that it was necessary to take action. She nourished herself by learning, by keeping up an active interest in a wide range of topics. She made a choice. She took responsibility for her life. She did not let "I can't" get in her way. She went out and did it.

Guidelines for Setting Goals

Goals are what keep you going. They should be:

Specific

Measurable

Limited in time

Attainable

Written down

Restated often

Start from Where You Are

A pattern of thought that can lock a person into stress begins, "If only . . ." *If only I had done this or hadn't done that, my life would be so much easier. If only I'd gone to college. If only I'd saved my money. If only I wasn't burdened with my sick mother. If only I would win the lottery.* This type of thinking blocks you from acting. Regrets and remorse don't move you forward an inch. To get anything done, you will have to start from right here, from where you are now. Accepting this fact is the first step in the road to accomplishment.

Sara did not waste time bemoaning her fate. She began from where she was. She heeded the old saying: *You'll never be any younger than you are today.*

VI Start From Where You Are— Don't Worry About the Past

Woodrow Wilson said: "We grow by dreams." Think about it. Everyone needs goals. To achieve wellness, you need a reason to get up every morning. You need something to work toward.

Take some time to look at your goals. Write them down.

Think about the steps that will get you there. Picture clearly in your mind where you're headed. Most importantly, make a plan to reach your goals.

It was a fine thing that Sara achieved her goal of a graduate degree. But what really made her special wasn't the degree, it was the process. It was her continual striving. It was her motivation. Her goals.

Awareness—

- Am I moving ahead right now, or stagnating?
- Am I quicker to look for reasons why I can't do something than to find ways that I can?
- Where do I want to be five years from now?

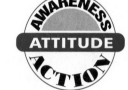

Attitude—

"I can start right now, today, to move toward the important goals in my life. Even the smallest step forward puts me closer."

Action—

Pick out something you've wanted to accomplish but have never gotten around to. Do something right away that will move you closer toward that goal.

Stop Procrastinating Now

One of the most common blocks to taking action is to keep putting things off. Here are some hints for getting things done:

1. Break up large tasks into small ones.
2. Focus on priorities.
3. Make a beginning even if you can go no further.
4. Don't wait for the "right" moment.
5. Work in short bursts.
6. Reward yourself for starting, finishing.
7. Set personal deadlines.
8. Accept imperfection.

Helping Others to Wellness

You are the type of person who cares about others, or you wouldn't be in emergency service. Once you've begun to climb the Staircase of Wellness, look around and see if you can't share some of what you've learned. We all know people, maybe those we work with, maybe family members, who are stuck at square one and are getting beaten up by stress.

The best way to help is by your example. Sara inspired the people she came in contact with. You don't need to preach. You just need to project the type of attitude that wellness generates.

You can share your experience:

"I didn't think I could kick the smoking habit, either. But I did it."

"I was pushing myself too hard. I decided I needed to create some time and space for myself."

"I used to let those things bug me until I blew up. But now I take a minute to step back and tell myself I'm in control."

If someone asks for advice, your message should be simple:

When stress builds, look at your Total Person. Work toward balance in all areas of your life.

Always keep moving toward greater wellness. Make the choices. Take action. Nourish yourself. And always tell yourself: I can.

SUMMARY

- The facets of your life are part of a Total Person.
- Stress spills over from one area to another.
- Wellness means looking at health as a continuum, not as a static condition.
- We need to continually take positive steps toward optimum wellness:

  Accept change as part of life.

  Take action now to deal with stressful situations.

  Nourish yourself in order to prevent future stress.

  Make choices and take responsibility for your life.

For Further Thought

1. Think about ways stress spills over: How does physical stress such as illness affect your mental readiness? What impact does a social loss, such as the break up of a relationship, have on the emotional and spiritual aspects of a person's life?

2. In what ways do we divide our lives into compartments? How might this aggravate stress?

3. Discuss how your EMS work might have given rise to stress in the five areas of your life: social, emotional, mental, physical, spiritual.

4. List three excuses a person suffering from overwhelming stress might give to avoid seeking professional help.

5. How does the concept of wellness differ from the traditional view of illness and health?

6. Name five events that you encounter in EMS that move you away from optimum wellness.

CHAPTER 5

The Power of the Mind

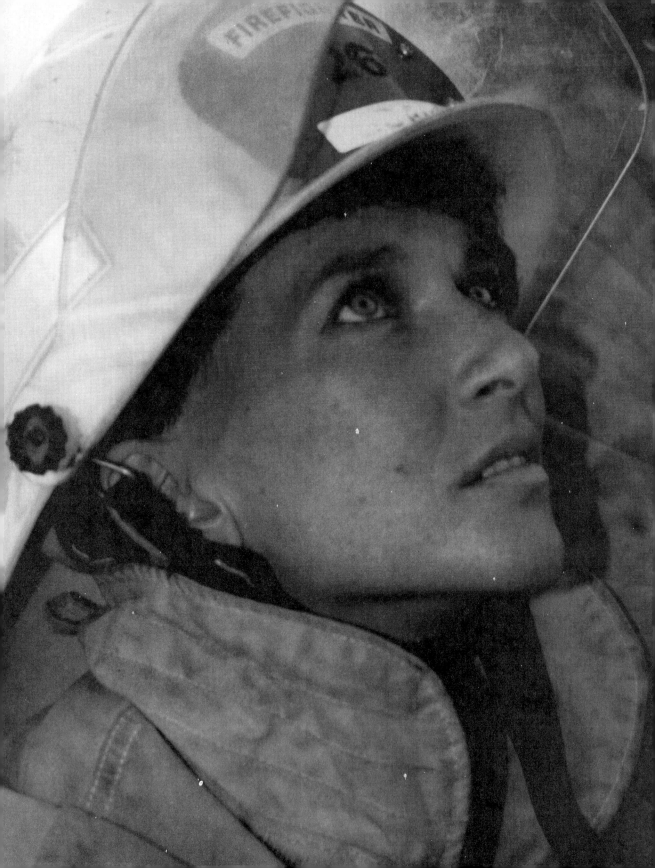

The Power of the Mind

An emergency room nurse told this story about a stressful incident:

"Toward the end of a busy shift I pick up the phone in the ER. It's the director of nursing. She tells me that the hospital review board has asked that I meet with them at 10 o'clock tomorrow morning.

"The words are barely out of her mouth when my palms begin to sweat and my chest tightens. I ask what they want. 'I'm not sure,' she says. 'They just told me to have you report to them.'

"Now my mind is racing. At first I can't imagine what it's about. Then I start going over every patient who's come through the ER during the last two months. I thought I'd given the best possible care, but maybe I slipped up. Maybe I said something and a patient took it the wrong way. Maybe someone's going to sue. Should I talk to a lawyer? I'm going to lose my job. My husband's depending on my income to meet the mortgage payments. What can I tell him? And how can I get another job with this on my record?

"The rest of the day was a blur. At home I couldn't eat, couldn't sleep. My husband asked me what was wrong. 'Nothing,' I said. He knew better.

"Driving to the hospital the next morning I almost had an accident. I kept thinking, 'My career is over. This is it.' When I sat down in front of the review board I could hardly keep my hands from shaking.

"The chairman of the review board opened by telling me that I was not the subject of their investigation. They simply wanted some input from me. I hardly heard the rest of what he said, I was so relieved that I wasn't going to lose my job. All that worrying for nothing."

This person underwent a good deal of genuine stress. What was the origin of it?

The Role of the Mind in Stress

Stressors, the events that cause stress, are out there in the world. In this case, the stressor was the request to report to the review board. Many of the symptoms of stress show up in the body—sweaty palms, shakiness, loss of appetite. But in between the two is that crucial link: **the mind.**

The mind generates stress by interpreting the stressful event. In some cases, the interpretation is correct. *"This situation is dangerous, I need to be alert."* At other times, as with this nurse, the interpretation is completely wrong. Right or wrong, it doesn't matter: the stress is the same.

Your body doesn't know whether your mind has interpreted the situation correctly. If the stressful thoughts are present, the body reacts. Unfortunately, the mind can take a completely neutral event and turn it into a negative stress reaction.

In this case, the nurse turned a summons from the review board into a scenario in which she would be sued, her career would go down the tubes, and she and her husband would lose their home. Logical? Sensible? No. But the point is: Logic doesn't matter. All that matters is what you believe. She reacted to the negative thoughts as if they were true.

It happens all the time. You get a notice of a tax audit. You've been scrupulous about your taxes, but it still keeps you up at night. Your spouse is a couple of hours late getting home from a trip. All of a sudden you're imagining the worst.

No one has ever died from taking an EMT final. But you'd think from the sleepless nights and nervous stomachs leading up to the test that it was a matter of life and death. What's happening? The mind is taking an event and turning it into a negative stressor.

Vanishing Fear

A man walking down a path encountered a poisonous snake ready to strike. He became terrified. He couldn't move. He thought he was facing death. Then he noticed that it wasn't a snake, it was an old piece of rope. Relieved, he walked happily on his way.

Question: What happened to this man's fear? Isn't it better to neutralize fears rather than overcome them? In some cases, a little more information changes the complexion of things entirely.

Or consider the phone call you receive at 3 a.m. Your heart is in your mouth as you pick up the receiver. The same phone rings at 3 p.m. and you're completely relaxed answering it. Why? In the first case you imagine an accident, the death of a loved one, some grave tragedy. In the second case you don't. The stimulus is the same. It's not just the stimulus that causes the stress. It's what you think and believe.

There's good news here, too. Each of us has the power to influence how we perceive events. Not only can we shut off the irrational negative thoughts that cause stress, we can also substitute positive, stress-reducing thoughts to help us deal with real problems and dangers in the world.

Irrational Beliefs

- I'm being called before the review board—I'm sure to lose my job.
- I made a mistake—I'm going to be sued.
- Joe didn't say hello to me—he hates me.
- I forgot my sister's birthday—I'm a bad person.
- The heart monitor is a complex instrument—I'll never be able to understand it.

These are examples of irrational beliefs. They are an important factor in creating the stress in our lives. Why? Because we react to the belief as if it were true. In most cases it isn't true, but we react anyway.

Common Irrational Beliefs

"You can't trust anyone."

"I'm a loser."

"I'll die if . . ."

"You can't teach an old dog new tricks."

"I failed so I'm worthless."

"I deserve this punishment."

"My life should always flow smoothly."

"I can't . . ."

Often we're not even aware of what we're thinking. Irrational, stress-producing thoughts are automatic. They may stem from a need to rehearse, to prepare for difficult events to come. They may simply result from our outlook on the world, a habit of negative thinking.

We're affected by many different types of irrational thoughts. Here are a few examples:

Personalization. You feel that events, particularly other people's actions, are directed at you. Betty may be frowning because she's trying to remember something—but you think, irrationally, that she disapproves of what you're doing.

Mind reading. You assume you know what people are thinking about you. You made a mistake on a call, so the whole squad is laughing at you.

Polarization. You see events in black and white terms, ignoring shades of gray. If it isn't perfect, it's lousy.

Generalization. You draw a broad conclusion from a single incident. "I failed a quiz, so I must be stupid. "

Awfulizing. You think the worst is bound to happen. The nurse described in the case study awfulized after being told to report to the review board.

A story is told about President John F. Kennedy. When he was a young congressman he was sitting with a friend discussing the play, "Brigadoon," which he'd just seen. An aide called and said that there was an unconfirmed report that Kennedy's sister had been involved in a plane crash. Kennedy's reaction: Call me back if it's confirmed. He went on talking about the musical. A few minutes later, the news was confirmed—his sister was dead. Kennedy broke into tears.

> *Assuming in advance that the worst will happen simply generates unnecessary stress.*

Call me back if it's confirmed—it's a good antidote against awfulizing and the other forms of irrational beliefs. The point is not that the worst never happens. Sometimes it does. When it does you will deal with it and you will cope. Assuming in advance that the worst will happen simply generates unnecessary stress.

Awareness—

- Get the facts. What's the actual event? Separate what is actually happening from what you are imagining. The nurse was told to report to the review board. Nothing more. That was the only fact available.

- Isolate the beliefs. "What am I telling myself?" Look closely at your irrational thoughts. "I'm going to be sued. I'll lose my job. My husband will hate me." These are not facts, only assumptions.

- Examine the effects. What are these thoughts doing to you? Are your thoughts making you nervous, anxious? Are they causing physical distress? Are they preventing you from functioning properly?

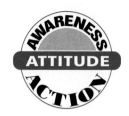

Attitude—

"I won't be stampeded into stress by irrational thoughts. I am in control of my thinking. To worry solves nothing."

Action—

Substitute positive thoughts for negative ones. "I'm a competent nurse. I can handle the situation. I'm confident about my abilities. There's nothing to worry about."

Watch Those Labels

It's often our labels that turn neutral events into stressors. A label implies a point of view. In your emergency work you regularly enter a situation that others label "a disaster" or "a crisis." As an emergency responder, you look on the same situation as a "manageable event," even a "routine call."

The labels you apply influence your attitude. They help determine your perspective on events.

One person sees a situation as a problem, another sees it as an opportunity. One sees an obstacle, the other sees a challenge. Which one is going to suffer more stress? Which is more likely to handle the situation successfully?

People we call handicapped now frequently refer to themselves as "challenged." Why? It puts their situation in a different light. Someone once said, *"In nature there are neither rewards nor punishments—there are consequences."* It's all a question of labels.

Feeling Good About Yourself

- Practice complimenting yourself often and with meaning.

- Do not allow others to diminish your self worth.

- Do not use external factors to measure your self worth.

The Power of Thoughts

All of us talk to ourselves all the time. We may be aware of it, usually we're not. Sometimes we take control of this inner monologue, but normally it continues on automatic pilot.

Your inner monologue includes statements about the world, about what's happening, about other people, and especially about yourself.

"I'm good at dealing with patients—I'm not mechanically inclined—I screwed up on that call last night—I've never been a good student—I'm a skillful driver—I'm afraid to express myself in meetings."

These thoughts affect you. To the subconscious, thoughts are as real as facts. Every statement you make registers in your subconscious. It isn't analyzed, it simply sinks in.

What happens? Your behavior begins to be influenced by your thoughts. You think you can't, so you can't. You don't even try. You tell yourself you're not mechanically inclined, so you never take the time to focus your attention on mechanical tasks. You tell yourself you're a bad student, so what's the point of studying? You tell yourself you're good at dealing with patients, so you approach patient care with confidence and a positive outlook that's contagious.

It's very important to become aware of how your inner monologue is contributing to your stress. Does it consist of a steady flow of irrational beliefs? Does it constantly hamper your efforts with negative thoughts?

You've heard of voodoo. There are recorded instances of people dying simply because they believed a curse had been put on them.

You've seen the power of thoughts in your EMS work. You suggest to a patient that they're going to be feeling better, and they do feel better. Why? Because you've influenced their inner monologue. Instead of "I *hurt*," they're thinking, "*The pain is easing.*"

Tune in to Your Inner Monologue

Take some time to tune in to your inner monologue: Sit in a comfortable chair. Spend a few minutes breathing easily, become aware of your breath flowing in and out. Try to keep the awareness on your breath as you turn your attention to your thoughts.

Your goal is not to suppress thoughts, but to avoid boarding a thought train. When a thought comes into your head tell yourself "I'm thinking," and let the thought go.

If you do find yourself caught up in an inner monologue simply stop, focus again on your breathing and start over.

Practice this technique for a few minutes every day, gradually increasing the time.

Tuning in to your inner monologue has two benefits. First, it makes you more aware of what you're thinking and how your thoughts contribute to stress. Second, it tends to be a relaxing process in itself. It gives you a short break, a time of inner quiet.

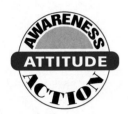

Awareness—

Consider the way in which thoughts influence how you act. You think, "I'm a shy person." You act shy. But is the thought a reflection of the reality? Or does the thought create the reality?

Attitude—

"I need not let my inner monologue determine my behavior. I can take control of it and use it to my advantage."

Action—

At random times during the day stop and ask yourself, *"What am I thinking? Have I been caught up in negative thoughts?"*

Affirm the Positive

Having considered your irrational beliefs and examined your inner monologue, you've become aware of the amount of stress that arises from negative thinking. Maybe you're assuming negatives that have no basis in fact. Maybe you're taking the negative things that happen every day and blowing them out of proportion in your mind. The result is the same: an increase in stress means a decrease in the positive energy you need to deal with the situations you face.

Consider the story of Bob, a 23-year-old volunteer firefighter:

"I had always been attracted to EMS work and hoped to eventually locate a job in emergency medicine and do it as a career. The problem was, I started having doubts about my ability to work with patients. I was afraid I wouldn't do the right thing. This fear kept growing even though I usually performed OK on the scene.

"But then it got so bad that I dreaded hearing the tones for an ambulance call. I would get so wound up that I couldn't make decisions. I couldn't think.

"I was at the point of giving up the whole thing when I decided to talk to a counselor. He told me to tune in to what I was telling myself.

"That wasn't so hard. I was telling myself, 'You've got a problem. You're afraid. You can't depend on yourself. You get nervous. Everybody knows you can't hack it.'

"I asked him how I could overcome my fear. He had a funny answer. 'You don't have to overcome it,' he said. 'You just have to replace your negative thoughts with positive ones.' He gave me a list of simple statements to make:

> *I'm in control.*
> *I welcome the challenge of each call.*
> *I think quickly under pressure.*
> *I make decisions and carry them through.*
> *I am effective when I'm on an ambulance call.*

"I memorized these statements and repeated them three times during the day, before going to bed, and whenever tones went off for a call. Just the repetition made me start to believe them.

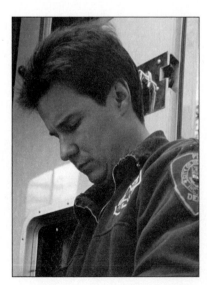

"At first I still felt some fear. But when I saw that I could operate effectively, the fear diminished. I knew I wasn't just fooling myself. I had every reason to think positively."

Affirmations are important for emergency responders because they help prevent stress from getting a grip on you. As you've already seen, it's far better to neutralize stress than to endure it or to deal with its effects on your life.

The Process of Affirmation

It's easy to decide to change a habit, attitude or situation. But deciding doesn't bring about the change. This is especially true when you're dealing with something as elusive as your thoughts. You need a specific process for creating the clear positive image that will replace and counteract the negative way you've been thinking.

The reason that some people give up on affirmations too soon is that the positive thoughts you create have to compete with the negative ones that are habitual. Say you're reluctant to contribute ideas at meetings. You create an affirmation: "*I am calm and confident when I speak up at meetings.*" You say it to yourself. Fine.

The problem is, you've said something different to yourself a thousand times: "*My ideas are no good. People don't want to hear them. I'll make a fool of myself.*" What will your subconscious believe? The message it's heard over and over.

You need to imprint your affirmation through frequent repetition. Every time you repeat it, you should do three things:

1. **State your affirmation with emotion.** Say it aloud when you can. "*I am calm and confident when I speak up at meetings.*"

2. **Picture the outcome you want as if it were already true.** See yourself speaking confidently.

3. **Take a minute to experience the feeling of the new behavior.** You've just presented your idea at a meeting—you've made a contribution. You're satisfied.

Repeat the affirmation frequently, but not just mechanically. Say it with feeling, with a positive emotion. Reflect on it briefly. Just before you go to bed and on waking are good times to go over your affirmation. These are times when you are particularly open to the effects of the statement and image.

The process of affirmation requires trust. You won't see results immediately. After all, you're trying to counteract years of negative thinking. But affirmations require very little effort. And the process does work if you give it time and stick with it. It's been proven. It's not magic. It simply builds on the principle that your subconscious believes what it's told—if it's told often enough.

It's important to avoid the New Year's Resolution Syndrome. That's where you tell yourself, *"I'm going to give up junk food beginning January 1."* Sure enough, New Year's Day comes, no more junk food. But by January 5 your subconscious is asking, *"Where's my Big Mac with a side order of fries? I love that stuff."* By the sixth, you're pigging out.

Why? The subconscious believes you to be a lover of junk food. It has plenty of evidence to support that belief. It encourages you to engage in behavior that matches the image it holds as reality.

The affirmation process is different. You tell yourself, *"I am a person who eats right. It's easy for me to avoid greasy food."* You repeat the affirmation. You picture yourself eating right. And gradually you find that you have no craving for a Big Mac. You pass on the fries. Why? Your behavior aligns with the image you've planted in your subconscious.

Creating Affirmations to Combat Stress

Follow these guidelines to create affirmations:

1. **Make it personal.** The statement is by you, for you. The affirmation is an "I" statement. It refers only to the things that are under your control—not to how others act.

   "I take pride in the way I dress."

   "I welcome the challenge of taking the advanced trauma course."

2. **Make it positive.** Make the affirmation a positive sentence. Don't describe what you're not—this will only remind your subconscious of the negatives you're try-

ing to eliminate. Don't create an affirmation like, "*I am no longer nervous when I start an IV.*" That puts the emphasis on your present nervousness. Instead declare, "*I am confident and skilled when I start an IV.*"

3. **Use the present tense.** Your subconscious is always in the present. Tomorrow has no meaning. You are affirming an image that exists now. Speak about actual achievement, not distant hopes. "*I am confident when I drive the ambulance.*" "*I am relaxed when I meet new people.*"

4. **Employ action and emotion.** Use words that describe you moving ahead with ease and confidence, free of anxiety. "*I enjoy…*" "*I find it easy to…*" "*I quickly and enthusiastically…*" "*I am capable of…*"

5. **Create a picture.** Your affirmation should be clear and specific. Make sure you can see the behavior you want to achieve. Picture it. Avoid an affirmation like, "*I'm going to become a better EMT.*" Instead, say something like, "*I enjoy reading up on current EMS information.*" Or, "*I take time to review my skills every week.*" These affirmations allow you to see yourself engaging in the behavior.

As an exercise, create an affirmation related to some aspect of your life that has been causing you stress. Write it down. Memorize it. Try repeating it at least a dozen times a day over the next week.

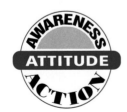

Awareness—

Negative statements affect my behavior in negative ways. What am I telling myself about myself?

Attitude—

"I can make positive changes by substituting affirmations for negative thinking. The effects will be beneficial if I make use of affirmations regularly."

Action—

Remember the formula of affirmation:
Say it—See it—Believe it—Become it.

Avoiding Life's Hooks

An EMT with a volunteer rescue squad told about an incident we can all relate to:

"I'm just sitting down to breakfast Saturday morning. I haven't had my coffee yet. Tones go out for an accident on the highway. I respond directly to the scene.

"I'm driving with my blue light flashing. About half a mile from my house, a car pulls out in front of me, the guy doesn't even look. I have to slam on my brakes to avoid rear-ending him. I give him the horn—he still doesn't glance in his mirror.

"The road has plenty of curves, there's nowhere to pass. He's driving at 30 mph thinking he's the only car on the road. I'm getting more and more angry by the minute, leaning on the horn.

"After a couple of miles, by which time I'm boiling over, he sees me. Does he pull off to the side? No. He just puts on his brakes, as if I'm supposed to pass him on a curve. So now we're going even slower. I could kill this guy. My heart is pounding, I'm grinding my teeth.

"Finally I take a chance, cross the double line, go by him. I floor it all the way to the scene. When I get there it turns out to be a fender-bender, no injuries. A good thing, because I'm way too irritated to be of much use anyway."

What's happening here? This man is suffering unnecessary stress because he's bitten at one of life's hooks. We encounter them every day. They're baited with all the annoyances that we sometimes call "pet peeves." In this case, the bait is incompetence. It might also be injustice, paperwork, noisy children, tardiness, anything you can think of.

Hooks are doubly dangerous when it comes to generating stress. To begin with, we react to them automatically and without thinking. We take the bait and find ourselves hooked on stress before we stop to consider. It becomes a habit.

Also, we often think that it's perfectly reasonable to swallow the hook. That driver who cuts you off without thinking *is* incompetent. He *deserves* the anger you feel. That's what you tell yourself. You feel justified in creating stress for yourself, so you do it over and over.

The fact is that the world is full of incompetence. But what does your reaction accomplish? You aren't educating someone by getting angry and blowing your horn at him. He doesn't even know you're there, most likely. He goes along on his merry way, leaving you to suffer the effects of the stress you've created.

Awareness is essential here. You've got to learn to see the hooks coming. This EMT should have recognized, as soon as the other car pulled out, that the situation was baited. Instead of laying on his horn, he should have slowed down, taken a deep breath, and talked to himself positively: *"This guy is incompetent, but I'm not letting it bother me. I'll get to the scene when I get there. I can't change this situation by becoming upset. I have more important things to think about."*

hooks The minor annoyances that a person reacts to automatically and repeatedly, contributing to overall stress.

Injustice

Life isn't fair. A paramedic told the story of coming to a police roadblock where the officers were checking inspection and registration stickers. She wasn't worried because hers were current. But the trooper asked her to pull to the side anyway.

"Ma'am," he said, "I'm going to write you a ticket. Seat belts are mandatory in this state and you're not wearing yours."

As she waited for him to fill out the ticket she watched the cars rolling by. It seemed like half the drivers weren't wearing seat belts. But the troopers were waving them on. She began to get angry. Why her? It wasn't fair. These people were doing the same thing and getting away with it.

But she was able to stop herself in time. She saw the image of the hook baited with injustice. She decided not to take it. It was bad enough having to pay the fine without making herself feel worse about it. Life isn't fair, what else is new? This would be a lesson always to wear her seat belt. Let it go at that.

What are your hooks?

Being ignored?

People who waste your time?

Bureaucracy and red tape?

Having to wait in line?

Being laughed at?

Unnecessary rules and regulations?

Incompetence?

Injustice?

Be on the look out for them. If you see them coming, you can prevent a lot of stress in your life. You will learn to react calmly and appropriately to situations that used to hook you and send you into a rage.

NOTE: Avoiding the hook that's inside issues like incompetence and injustice doesn't mean you ignore the situation or sit back and do nothing. Real incompetence can be dangerous, especially on the scene of an emergency. Real injustice exists and needs to be addressed. But getting worked up about it never helps. The more angry you get, the less likely you are to take the appropriate action to correct the situation. Your motto should be:

Don't get mad or get even—get smart.

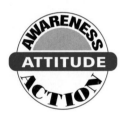

Awareness—

- What things make me furious without thinking?
- What are my pet peeves?

Attitude—

"I don't need to respond. I can prevent these hooks from taking over and causing me unnecessary stress."

Action—

1. Make a list of the three things that most often hook you into stress. Remember the times you've bitten at these hooks, and the feelings that resulted.
2. When you see the hook coming, label it. Say to yourself, "Injustice" or, "Incompetence."
3. Step back from the situation. Don't do anything for the time it takes to breathe deeply three times.
4. Get the facts straight. What's really going on here?
5. Talk to yourself. Use the process of affirmation described above.
6. If the situation can't be resolved and you find yourself getting upset, walk away. Better to retreat than to bite the hook.

A Positive Approach to Anger

Anger often plays a large role in stress, and emergency responders are no exception. At the scene of an auto accident you find that a drunk driver has severely injured several people. It makes you angry. You're a volunteer rushing to a call on a cold winter night, and the patient complains all the way to the hospital about the slow service. It burns you up.

Sometimes we think of anger as a bad emotion. It isn't. Anger is a valid emotion and you have every right to feel angry. Anger is a physical and emotional arousal that sends a message: something is bothering you.

But anger is a difficult emotion to handle. If you suppress it, it tends to fester. It can become a big factor in contributing to all the negative effects of stress, from headaches to heart disease. If you express your anger inappropriately, in a rage or a tantrum, the resulting aggression can taint your relationships and tear down your self-esteem.

Not all anger is justified. Blaming a person for an honest mistake or for something over which they have no control is unfair. Getting angry over an inanimate object—your car when it won't start in the morning—is pointless. But you can express just anger when a person knowingly, intentionally, and unnecessarily acts in a hurtful manner.

Expressing Anger

There are several ways not to express anger.

- Don't keep it bottled up, then let it out to your spouse or someone else who's not responsible for it. Learn to express your anger in a loving way. Allow it to teach the offender, to help that person to understand why you are upset. Work toward a resolution of the problem.

- Don't seek relief from anger in cigarettes, alcohol, or an eating binge.

- Don't turn to self-destructive behavior in order to demonstrate your displeasure.

Try replacing these unhealthy and unproductive expressions of anger with the following techniques:

- When you're angry with a person, tell them so. Get together with them later to talk. Make sure you say exactly how you felt and why you were angry. Try to include something positive about the incident—how it might have been done. Focus on the incident or the behavior, and not on the person. Emphasize that it's what the person did that made you angry. Then listen, let the other person talk.

- Don't pass up the opportunity to express your anger. Suppressing it and accepting behavior that makes you mad is likely to fill you with tension that will surface as stress symptoms later.

If your problem is expressing your anger too freely, you can take a number of steps to keep your cool:

- Be alert for the arousal that culminates in anger.

- When you feel yourself becoming angry, try to keep task-oriented. That is, focus on what you want to accomplish, not on simply letting out your anger.

- Assert yourself, but don't create unnecessary antagonism.

- Tell yourself that you are in control, that you don't need to give in to your anger.

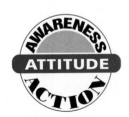

Awareness—

Anger is a tricky emotion to handle. You need to be alert to what makes you angry and how you deal with your feelings.

Attitude—

"I have every right to feel angry, but I'm not going to let anger control me. I will use my anger to accomplish what I want to do."

Action—

If anger is a problem, keep an anger journal. Record with whom you become angry and to whom you express it. Note how long you stay angry, what thoughts come to you, and what the result of your anger is. Look for patterns.

Anger as a Cue

The feelings of anger you feel should act as a cue to set off certain thoughts and actions. When you notice yourself becoming angry:

Think: "I have a right to be angry, but I'm going to keep it under control."

Act by remaining focused on the task. What can you get out of this situation by expressing your anger in a controlled way?

Handling Anxiety

You're familiar with the adrenaline "rush" that comes when you respond to an emergency. You may label it "nerves" or "excitement." It's a normal, healthy reaction. It gears you up for action. It puts you in a state of alertness. It provides a burst of energy.

But sometimes this feeling gets out of control. It turns into anxiety. You become so nervous that you can't function properly. You can't achieve the distance you need to keep events in perspective. You become physically shaky. Instead of clarifying your thoughts, anxiety can make your mind go blank. Anxiety has four distinct phases:

1. **Anticipation.** This is exaggerated worry before an event. It stems from fear of the unknown. Tomorrow you have to take your recertification exam. You dwell on it, think about all it stands for, and grow increasingly nervous.

Or maybe you've just been elected an officer in your rescue squad. You have no experience at taking charge of a scene. You're not sure how you'll perform. You imagine all that could go wrong.

2. **Confrontation.** An even more intense anxiety may take over as you come face to face with the situation you've been worrying about. You sit down to take the test. You head out on the ambulance to the first scene you will be in command of. All your uncertainties come to a head. The natural effect of adrenaline makes your anxiety worse.

3. **Action.** You are actually involved in what you have dreaded. Your earlier anxiety might increase your doubts about your abilities. You struggle to keep yourself under control.

4. **After the fact**. Sometimes the anxiety stays with you. It takes the form of endlessly reviewing what you did, what the outcome was. You worry about answers you gave to test questions even though there's no way to change them. You worry about how you handled a call.

The key to handling anxiety is to remain task-oriented. We've all had the experience in which we spent more time worrying about a test than we did studying for it. With a task-orientation you put your energy into actions that will maximize your performance. Before the exam, review the skills you are least sure of. Before you take over as squad officer, read through your squad's operating procedures so you'll be more confident. Most important: do something.

> *The key to handling anxiety is to remain task-oriented.*

Distance is another important way to deal with anxiety. Find activities that put the event out of your mind. Often it's a good idea to take a long walk or go out to a movie the night before a test or a job interview. Don't dwell on it.

Positive statements can be very helpful for dealing directly with all forms of anxiety. Normally you will be flooded with negative images, imagining the worst.

Combat their effects by substituting positive thoughts:

Anticipation

"Worry changes nothing."
"I will be able to do what's needed."
"I am in control. I know my stuff."

Confrontation

"I can take charge and get this done."
"I am focused on what I'm doing."
"I am relaxed and breathing deeply."

Action

"I'm doing this the best I can."
"I have everything under control."
"Soon I will have accomplished my goal."

After the fact

"I did it as well as I could have."
"I learned from this experience."
"This proved I don't need to worry."

Awareness—

- What situations cause me to feel anxiety?
- What is the effect of worrying and feeling anxious?

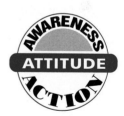

Attitude—

"My thoughts create the anxiety I feel. I can get a grip on these feelings by remaining task oriented. I can perform well even if I feel a little nervous."

Action—

Sometimes anxiety causes the train of our thoughts to take us places we don't want to go. We almost seem to be prisoners of our own minds as thoughts tumble one after another.

You can bring this intense worry under control. The technique is called **Thought Stopping**. All it requires is the initial awareness that you are engaging in inappropriate negative thinking.

You say out loud: "Stop!" If the thought continues, say it again. Shout it if necessary.

Later you will be able to cut off a train of thought simply by thinking "Stop."

Creating A Script for Success

Many top athletes prepare for important events by creating a success script. For example, a tennis player goes over an entire match in his head before going out onto the court. He sees himself performing well, anticipates any problems that might arise, and visualizes the outcome. This creates a script that aids his performance at difficult times during the match.

Turn the power of your mind to your advantage.

Scripting helps turn the power of your mind to your advantage. It can be particularly useful to prepare for difficult calls. For example, imagine a school bus accident with multiple injuries. You are the first one on the scene. Go over in your mind what you would do. Try to think how you will feel, what distractions and problems will arise. Move through the call in a detailed, step-by-step manner.

Scripting can be used to build confidence in many situations. If you have a problem with a particular skill—applying a traction splint, for example—visualize yourself going through the application steps in detail. If you're uncomfortable with auto extrication, create scripts for a number of different types of accidents.

The situation in the real world won't exactly correspond to your script. You'll have to improvise. The script will provide the basic pattern of behavior, which you can adapt to the conditions you find.

Some hints for effective scripting:

- Include every step. Don't skip over part of the procedure.
- See it happening in your mind. Visualize as clearly as you can.
- Anticipate problems so you're not frustrated when they happen. Someone has left the straps off the head immobilizer. What do you do?
- Always carry the script through to a successful conclusion.

Mental Defense Against Stress

It's not reassuring to imagine that your own mind is working to create stress in your life. But you've seen how it happens. Don't think to yourself: *"If I can't control my own thoughts, I'm really in trouble."*

Instead, take the attitude: *"The fact that my mind generates much of my stress means that I have control over it."*

Recognize that you can choose. You can go with the negative thoughts that have always increased your stress and hampered your efforts. Or you can substitute positive, stress-reducing thoughts that boost your confidence and performance. You are in charge.

Awareness—
- How do my thoughts affect me?
- Are some of my ideas and beliefs about myself irrational?

Attitude—
"I am not a chronic worrier. I can stop unnecessary worry and anxiety."

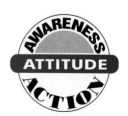

Action—

Here are some specific things you can do to use your mind to fight stress rather than add to it:

1. **Break down events.** Don't let them overwhelm you. Deal with them step by step. At each step, examine what you're thinking. What are your assumptions? Are they rational?

2. **Write your thoughts.** Many ideas appear sensible until we write them down. Then we immediately recognize them as irrational. Write down both the negative thoughts that add to stress and the positive affirmations that will replace them. A journal can be an excellent tool for recognizing the negative aspects of your thinking.

3. **Talk about what you think.** You may find that others in your squad share many of the same illogical ideas and thoughts that you do.

4. **Reward your success.** Whenever you resist taking the bait that you know contains the hook of stress, give yourself a small reward. When positive thinking works for you, tell yourself that you've made progress.

SUMMARY

- The mind plays a crucial role in creating negative stress reactions.

- Many of the beliefs we hold about ourselves are irrational.

- Examples of irrational thinking include:

  Personalization   Generalization
  Mind reading   Awfulizing
  Polarization

- Labels play a role in shaping our thinking and creating stress.

- The inner monologue is the steady flow of thoughts in a person's mind.

- Affirmations are a powerful tool for changing behavior and reducing stress.

- We can avoid unnecessary stress by recognizing and rejecting life's hooks.

- Anger is a valid emotion, but it must be handled carefully to keep it from creating stress.

- The best way to deal with worry and anxiety is by staying task-oriented.

Labels Can Cause Stress

Stress-Producing	Stress-Reducing
Difficulty	Challenge
Disaster	Complication
Crisis	Opportunity
Obstacle	Learning experience
Defeat	Setback
Work	Fun
Failure	Achievement
Overworked	Busy
"I have to…"	"I want to…"
Getting old	Growing
Stressful	Exciting
Nervous	Alert

For Further Thought ————————

1. Think of a time when negative thinking caused you unnecessary stress. What were the facts as you knew them? What were the irrational beliefs involved? How did they affect you? What would you tell yourself if the event occurred right now?

2. Some people take the approach: "If I worry about it, it won't happen." Does this make sense?

3. A placebo is a pill that has effects even though it has no active ingredients. It works because the patient thinks it will work. Can you cite some other examples in which the power of the mind accomplishes real results?

4. List the three most common sources of stress in the emergency response field. For each one, write down an affirmation that would help reduce the stress.

5. List your own affirmations. Include both personal and EMS goals that you want to achieve.

6. Most of us have one particular hook that we always fall for. Name the one that gives you the most stress. Give an example of a time it "hooked" you.

CHAPTER 6

Critical Incident Stress

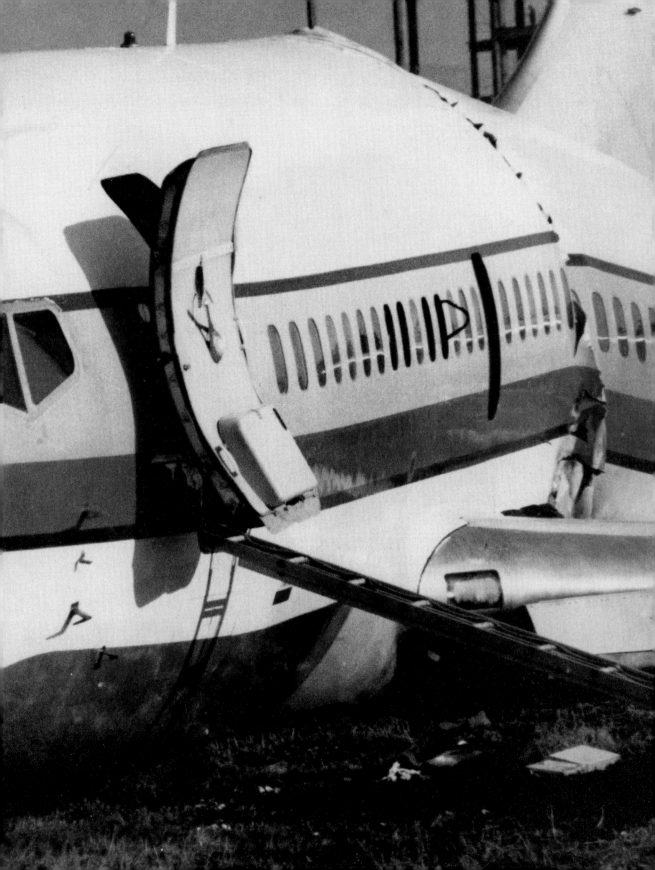

Critical Incident Stress

As an emergency responder you live a life marked by crisis. You regularly undergo experiences that an ordinary person might never encounter in a lifetime. You are trained to respond to these events in a calm and controlled manner, not to panic or to turn away.

You handle critical incidents as a professional, doing the things that need to be done. But it's important to take a professional attitude toward yourself as well. The stress that a critical incident generates is a danger to your well-being. It's a danger that you must take just as seriously as any other hazard you face in the field. If you don't, the repercussions of the event can threaten your mental and physical health. And the effects can linger for months or even years after the incident occurs.

The best way to defuse the stress that a critical incident can cause is for the rescuer to talk about what happened and how he or she feels, not try to hold feelings in.

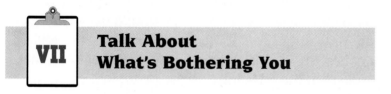

**VII   Talk About
What's Bothering You**

What is a Critical Incident?

The term critical incident often brings to mind images of disaster: a school bus down a ravine, a train derailment, a serious multi-vehicle accident, a house fire with multiple casualties, a plane crash.

Certainly these types of disasters are the most common category of critical incidents. The number of victims and the severity of their injuries creates a situation of peak urgency and emotional intensity.

critical
incident Any
situation faced by an
emergency service person
that causes him or her
to experience unusually
strong emotional
reactions, or overwhelms
the individual's ability to
cope and function.

But the real definition of critical incident is more personal. It's the situation that creates overwhelming stress in a particular emergency responder, stress that may prevent that person from functioning at the scene or later. An incident that's just another call for one person can be critical for another. Each of us brings a different personality and background to emergency service. Circumstances affect each of us differently.

Here are a few of the factors that can turn a routine call into a critical incident:

Incidents involving children. Every emergency responder knows that treating injuries or severe illnesses in children can be much more stressful than handling the same situations in adults. We all are affected by the innocence and helplessness of young victims. Parents immediately think of their own children. The death of a child is particularly difficult and can have a profound impact on the rescuers involved.

Trapped victims. A group of volunteer rescuers told the story of being called to an accident on a bad stretch of road. A tanker full of gasoline had gone down an embankment. The driver was trapped in the cab, severely injured. Gasoline had spilled, pooling all around the wreck. There was no way they could begin extrication until the spill was cleaned up. A single spark would have set off a major explosion. The driver died before they could get to him.

"Personally," one rescuer said, *"I would've given anything to save that guy."*

Even when rescuers can begin extrication immediately, the distress that a trapped victim feels can be contagious. The time required to free the person is frustrating. Sometimes rescuers must wait for additional equipment to arrive. Crucial decisions are required. All of this adds significantly to stress and can, for some, turn the situation into a critical incident.

Line-of-duty deaths or injuries. To have one of your colleagues killed or severely injured is devastating for most emergency responders. Besides being a deep personal loss, a line-of-duty death shatters the expectations that EMS people have about themselves—they are always the caregivers; it's the others that have the accidents and illnesses.

An incident involving a relative or close friend. Treating someone close to you can easily turn a routine call into a critical incident. Suddenly the professional distance that you are normally able to maintain when you are providing care evaporates.

Violence. Both the threat of violence on the job and the necessity of treating the results of violence can contribute to stress. Violence resulting in death or serious injury is disturbing. Having to operate in a hostile or potentially violent environment significantly adds to the pressure on rescue workers.

Distraught relatives. One of the most stressful tasks that an EMS worker faces is to deal with the emotionally upset relatives of a patient. Often this is doubly difficult because the need to comfort a bystander conflicts with patient care. In the case of a sudden death, relatives may turn to emergency responders for solace. Or they may vent their anger at emergency personnel, even hold them responsible for their relative's death. Any contact with distraught relatives puts an added burden on rescue workers.

Media attention. Just the presence of cameras and reporters can make rescuers feel they are operating under the critical eye of public attention. Reporters are sometimes insensitive and intrusive. For those who are not accustomed to it, media attention or the sometimes distorted accounts of an incident in the papers or on television can be very stressful.

Facing the "Big One"

Everyone who works in emergency service sooner or later encounters incidents that create extraordinary stress. An inexperienced EMT might worry that almost any call could be the **"big one."** Once they've been working in the field for a while, emergency responders sometimes swing the other way, become overconfident that they can handle any situation that comes their way without a problem. But truly experienced people know that there are going to be incidents that get to you. It doesn't matter how much you've seen or how hardened you think you've become.

The following are the commonly accepted examples of critical incidents:

A line-of-duty death.

A serious injury in the line of duty.

The suicide of a peer.

A mass-casualty incident.

The death or serious injury of a child.

An incident in which the victim is known to the rescuer.

A prolonged incident with a negative outcome.

Night operations.

Intense media interest surrounding an incident.

Dealing with the results of violence or operating in a violent environment.

A highway patrol officer, who's also an EMT, had worked on the expressway for 20 years. He'd seen every type of accident imaginable, all kinds of death. He told about responding to an accident at five in the morning on a heavily traveled section of highway.

"That stretch of road usually means a bad accident. Coming around the corner I saw smoke and realized we had a working car fire. At the scene we encountered a head-on crash. The van was fully involved. The trailer it was pulling had impacted the rear, rupturing the gas tank. I knew there were people inside, but I couldn't get close enough to help.

"The driver of the van was sitting on the road—somebody had pulled him out. He told me his wife, baby daughter, and son were inside, along with another couple. The fire department was on the scene quickly. They were able to get the baby out. I started to work on her. She was barely conscious, burned real bad. I kept hearing a faint little whimper. There wasn't much I could do except maintain an airway, give her oxygen, and pray the ambulance would arrive quickly. It did.

"I felt weak. I kept hearing that baby's little cry. I never experienced anything like it before. I was beaten by it. I remember feeling that I just wanted to crawl into bed and not have to see this anymore. At home I couldn't sleep.

"I can't understand why this one got to me. I thought I was losing my mind. I kept seeing the image of the accident, of that baby, kept hearing her cry over and over. Why this one?"

The point here is that this officer felt that he'd seen it all, that this incident was no worse than many others he'd encountered in the past.

What he failed to recognize was that no one is immune to critical incident stress. This scene presented him with a number of stress elements: multiple trapped victims, severe injury to a child, the emotional demands of dealing with a survivor. Added to these was the fact that he'd just worked a series of midnight shifts. Perhaps other stressors were affecting his life as well.

Everyone enters emergency service expecting to become involved from time to time in intense and tragic events. In the course of our work, we develop many coping mechanisms that allow us to function in the face of tragedy and chaos. Without these mechanisms we wouldn't be able to do our jobs.

But it's important to keep in mind that anyone's defenses can be overwhelmed. Every time you go out on a call, you may suddenly find yourself faced with the "big one." Maybe it's a scene you've encountered many times before. Today it gets to you.

Critical Incident Stress is Normal

At the scene of a major plane crash an EMT was discovered wandering among the trees, soaked from the rain, without a jacket. When an on-scene peer counselor approached him, the man was dazed and confused. Later the counselor said,

"This EMT had been in the main section of the cabin. He was working with a 14-year-old boy. The boy was pinned in his seat, buried under wreckage, still conscious. The EMT spent 45 minutes with him. He promised to get him out and reunite him with his father, who'd been removed earlier.

"The extrication proceeded slowly. The EMT kept hold of the boy's hand the whole time. He was still holding it when the boy died. The EMT removed his jacket, covered the child's body, exited the craft, and began to walk.

"When I found him, he was literally walking into trees. He was wet and cold, he didn't know where he was. I led him to a rescue truck and stayed with him. After a while he began to talk about what happened. He kept saying, 'I let him down. I should have been able to get him out. I let him down.' He broke into tears."

This EMT's reaction was entirely normal. That doesn't mean that everyone reacts the same to the same incident, or that a given person will be overwhelmed in the same way by a similar set of circumstances. But to be deeply affected by an incident is not a sign of weakness or failure or mental illness.

critical incident stress A normal stress reaction to a powerful negative event that overwhelms a person's ability to cope.

Remember the fact that is the basis for understanding stress in emergency service: Behind your role as an emergency responder is a Total Person. That person is human, with the full range of human emotions.

Firefighters can enter burning buildings because they wear protective gear—the Nomex, the vapor barrier, the Scott pack. But if the heat becomes intense enough, it overwhelms this protection. Safety requires an understanding that underneath that protective gear is a vulnerable human being.

Emergency responders, through their training and experience, develop psychological protective gear. These defenses allow them to face situations that would be too much for untrained individuals. But on any given call a rescue worker can encounter an incident so powerful that it overwhelms his or her defenses.

To be deeply affected by an incident is not a sign of weakness or failure or mental illness.

Awareness—

Any time you're out on a call that affects you in a way that other calls haven't, you should monitor yourself for stress reactions. This applies even if you've been on similar calls in the past.

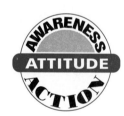

Attitude—

"The fact that I react strongly to some of the intense and tragic events I encounter is simply a sign that I'm a normal human being."

Action—

Talk about it. We will come back to this advice again and again in this chapter. Talk to one of your peers, your spouse, your unit's chaplain, a counselor, a friend. Talk about what happened, what you felt, how it's affecting you.

Cumulative Stress and Critical Incidents

You know how stress can accumulate in your life, often from a number of different sources, and sometimes without you being aware of it. That type of pressure can cause stress reactions even if you never face a critical incident. Likewise, a very powerful incident—a bad fire or severe auto accident—can overwhelm your defenses in a very direct way, as it did in the case of the EMT at the plane crash.

Often the two types of stress interact. Consider what happened to a veteran firefighter.

"I can't understand it," he told a counselor. "I could always put it behind me. Why not now? This call was a simple cardiac arrest. We worked on the guy for about 20 minutes. He died—most of them do. I've seen lots of people die. Never bothered me. But this one did. That night I kept seeing his face. Kept going over the call. It was like instant replay. I thought I was losing my mind. The incident kept nagging at me.

"I never thought I would need to talk to someone about the stress of the job. I've been around here 18 years. I've done all the tough jobs. But I've been seeing this guy's face for a week, not sleeping well, not wanting to go to work. I need an answer. Why now?"

As this man talked with the counselor, a number of additional facts came out. The cardiac call was the fifth in 10 days—all the patients died. On the last day of his tour his engine had been the first on the scene of a working house fire. Somebody yelled that there was a child in the house. This man had entered the fully involved structure to search. Fortunately the neighbor was mistaken, no one was home. The incident took its toll nevertheless.

In addition, the man was financing two daughters in college. He was working a part-time job to bring in extra income. He had little time to spend with his wife and family.

140

What happened? His defenses had been worn down by the cumulative stress in his life. A single incident suddenly became the one that overwhelmed him. His reaction was normal. No matter how many similar calls he'd responded to, this one became for him a critical incident, his "big one."

How Do I Know It's the "Big One?"

It should be clear by now that it isn't just the magnitude of the event itself that turns it into a critical incident. Even a routine call can turn into the "big one" for a given individual.

Awareness is important here. Critical incident stress can overwhelm you much more quickly than the cumulative stress of your daily routine. You need to be on the lookout for the symptoms and be ready to take quick action.

Short-Term Symptoms

These can occur during or immediately after the incident. If they aren't dealt with, they may also become long-term symptoms.

- **Visual or auditory distortions.** A police officer forced to shoot someone might report that he actually sees the bullet leave his gun. Rescuers in an intense situation might hear sounds as if from the end of a tunnel.

- **A feeling of unreality.** This can occur during a critical incident and may recur afterwards.

- **Time distortions.** Rescuers may think they've been working at a scene for 10 minutes when in fact an hour has passed. Events may seem to be happening in slow motion—or fast forward.

- **Emotional numbness.**

- **Confusion or disorientation.** Sometimes rescuers forget where they are.

- **Physical sensations.** Feelings ranging from dizziness and fatigue to difficulty breathing, elevated heart rate, or nausea.

- **Flashbacks of the critical incident.** This is a common symptom. Almost any stimulus can trigger a flashback in which the person finds himself or herself reliving the event.

- **Guilt and remorse.** The person may accuse himself of failing even when he did everything possible.

- **A sudden need to withdraw from contact with other people.**

- **Errors in judgement or mistakes in routine procedures.**

- **Anger and irritability.**

These, as well as many of the other signs of stress, can affect a person at the scene or soon afterward. It's crucial to be on the lookout for these symptoms in yourself and your colleagues during any high-pressure incident. Immediate intervention, even just removing the person from duties at the scene of a prolonged emergency, can help prevent long-term stress reactions. In addition, a rescuer who is being overwhelmed in this way can become a danger to himself and others.

Long-Term Symptoms

All of the signs and symptoms of stress that you read about in Chapter 3 can apply to critical incident stress reactions. Here are some of the ones to be on the lookout for in the days and weeks after the event:

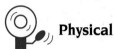 **Physical**

Fatigue and difficulty sleeping.

Headaches or unusual muscular aches or tremors.

Weakness, dizziness or sweating.

Difficulty breathing or hyperventilation.

Stomach problems, including nausea, diarrhea and indigestion.

Reduced sex drive, avoidance of intimacy.

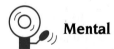 **Mental**

Intrusive images, flashbacks, intense memories of the sights, sounds and smells of the event.

An inability to concentrate.

Difficulty making decisions, doing calculations, solving problems.

Obsessive thoughts—the person may continually go over the details of the critical event.

Excessively heightened alertness.

Frequent nightmares.

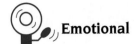 **Emotional**

Feelings of guilt or remorse.

Numbness or excessive detachment.

Intense anger.

Depression, feelings of intense grief. One EMT, who had performed CPR on a dying infant, stated afterward that he felt he had peered through a crack at the sadness that lies just below the surface of the world.

Loss of emotional control.

Fear, anxiety or apprehension.

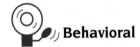 **Behavioral**

Intensified startle reflex.

Avoidance of things associated with the event. Some rescuers become reluctant to go on any call in the weeks after a crisis.

Changes in eating, working or other habits.

Isolation, withdrawal from social relationships.

Dependence on alcohol or drugs. Excessive smoking or eating are also common.

A desire not to be touched.

Destructive or high-risk behavior.

Becoming unusually quiet. Alternatively, the person may engage in nonstop talking as a barrier against emotional turmoil.

The symptoms of critical incident stress will most often emerge in the first few weeks after the incident. But it's important to understand that they can also affect a person long after the event.

A suburban police officer told this story:

"My buddy was a very experienced officer. He was assigned to car 306. He went out to start his shift one evening. An hour went by and car 306 wasn't responding to calls. I was just getting off and saw the cruiser still in the parking lot. The engine was running, the lights on. My friend was sitting behind the wheel. He didn't look at me. I went over, opened the door, touched his shoulder. He sort of woke up. I asked him what the matter was.

"He said he'd just relived an incident that happened exactly a year earlier. A car with 10 kids packed inside had tried to run a railroad crossing. A train plowed into them, demolished the car. Only one of them survived. 'I was there,' he told me. 'I saw, heard and smelled everything, just as if I was on that scene again. It was eerie.'"

Actually, it wasn't that strange. Anniversaries often trigger stress reactions. Holidays can have a similar affect. And it may take even less to bring back a flood of memories, something as simple as a smell can trigger the recurrence of images even years after an event.

Stress Defense at the Scene

When we're working at a critical incident, no matter what the circumstances, we're usually too involved in doing what needs to be done to be overcome by stress. We translate everything into action. But it's important to recognize that stress can take hold even during an event. This is especially true during prolonged disasters when fatigue overcomes the initial rush of adrenaline.

The mental and physical stress that a critical incident can generate are a safety factor as well. Stressed individuals are prone to mistakes and lapses of concentration.

Tunnel vision is also a problem, with rescuers ignoring obvious hazards in their rush to get the job done.

Both officers and individual rescuers on the scene should keep aware of the potential effects of stress and take action to prevent excessive stress before it occurs.

Here are some of the things that can be done:

☑ Keep a watch for any rescuer who is being overwhelmed by the stress of the incident. Erratic behavior, confusion or an outburst of emotion are a few of the signs. Such a person should be given an immediate rest break.

☑ Everyone should rest at least once every two hours. A break of half an hour is ideal.

☑ Rotation of duties helps to combat stress.

☑ Rescuers should take advantage of breaks to remove themselves from extreme heat or cold and to spend some time in a quiet place away from the scene.

☑ All emergency personnel should drink plenty of water during a disaster. The rule is: Drink before you are thirsty.

☑ A well-organized scene with clear lines of command is an important factor in reducing on-scene stress. Rescuers should be briefed before deployment if possible and should know what their duties are.

☑ Provisions should always be made at the scene to demobilize rescuers when they are finished with their jobs. Rather than going right home, they should spend 30-45 minutes winding down from the emotional intensity of the event. During this time it's a good idea to wash up, have something to eat, finish up any paperwork or reports, and receive information from line officers regarding debriefings.

☑ Immediately after a critical incident light physical exercise helps a person to unwind and counteracts some of the physical aspects of stress.

☑ It may also be helpful for rescuers to write down their thoughts and feelings when they get home from a disaster. This begins the process of organizing events and provides perspective.

Coping with Critical Incidents

One of the great things about emergency service is the sense of family that connects the people who work in the field. We laugh together, hurt together, and save lives together. It's important to keep in mind, when the "big one" hits, that you aren't alone. The people beside you may well be experiencing feelings very similar to your own. They can often provide you with the support and understanding that you need in a crisis.

An EMT who worked for a volunteer fire department told this story of a critical incident that his department went through a few years back:

"It was a house fire that took the lives of an entire young family, mom, dad, two kids. Despite our best efforts, the enemy, fire, won the battle. Every one of our members who were at the scene was troubled by this very powerful event. Without exception every one locked his or her feelings inside. Each of us thought we were alone in what we were feeling.

"We had a very perceptive chief who soon realized that his people weren't acting right. We were quieter than usual, isolated. We were often irritable with each other. We became reluctant to respond to calls. Some of us were drinking more than before. The chief realized that something needed to be done. He called on a stress debriefing team to come in and conduct a session at the fire house.

"No one was sure what to expect. The leader of the debriefing team explained that events such as this tragic house fire create many different reactions in participants. He told us that the best way to put the incident in perspective was to talk about it, to talk about what we were experiencing. He asked everyone present to honor the privacy of everyone else—what was shared in that room would stay in the room. We trusted each other on calls—we had to trust each other to share the pain that resulted.

"What was most surprising to all of us was the fact that many of our private thoughts, feelings and reactions to this event were shared by others. It was a relief just knowing that what we were feeling was normal, that we weren't alone."

One member said that the fire left him feeling very angry. He couldn't explain why, and he wasn't sure it was an appropriate feeling. But another firefighter spoke up and said he felt angry too. In fact, anger is a very normal reaction to an extremely stressful incident.

Other members talked about seeing vivid images of the fire over and over. Some had had problems sleeping. Still others talked about how it had made them appreciate their own families more. "I went home and hugged my kids," one said.

The debriefing team went on to explain stress reactions and to teach the rescuers techniques for handling the stress that any incident like this will generate. They answered the firefighters' questions.

During the debriefing session the entire mood in the room lifted. The incident would never be forgotten, but it ceased to have the powerful effect on the members of the department. It had been moved, in their minds, to a safer place.

The Debriefing Process

The idea of critical incident stress debriefing, or CISD, is threefold. First, to defuse the powerful emotions generated by a critical incident so that they do not cause short-term or long-term problems for rescuers. Second, to educate emergency people about stress reactions and how to handle them. Third, to identify and extend professional help to those individuals who have been so overwhelmed by the event that they are unable to cope.

The debriefing process is not easy. Reliving a difficult event and facing the intense feelings it generates can be very painful. It requires courage and trust. But what is accomplished during the one to three hours that it takes is very important.

Critical incident stress reactions are much easier to prevent than they are to treat later. When you transport a patient with a deep laceration the emergency room doctor doesn't just suture the cut closed. That would be an invitation to infection. First the wound must be cleaned and sterilized. The purpose of debriefing is to prevent hidden emotions from festering and coming out later in the form of stress reactions.

An additional benefit is that the debriefing brings the group of rescuers together into a tighter and more trusting relationship that benefits all. It highlights the bonds that join us together, and assures us that we have a group of supportive and understanding colleagues who can help us through the bad times.

Many of the concepts and techniques of CISD have been developed by Dr. Jeffrey Mitchell, who founded the International Critical Incident Stress Foundation to continue research and the application of debriefings in the field. Mitchell's ideas have reversed the old notion that the best way to react to a critical incident was to "tough it out." That approach never worked and was always an invitation to long-term stress problems.

critical incident stress debriefing (CISD) A psychological, emotional, and educational process to mitigate the impact of a critical incident on the rescuers involved.

Important: Keep in mind that a CISD session is not a critique or fact-finding meeting, nor do such meetings take the place of CISD.

The Debriefing Team

A debriefing team is usually headed by a mental health professional who has received specialized training in the stress of emergency service work. Often this person may have actual experience working as a paramedic or firefighter.

The team will also consist of several peer counselors. These are members of the emergency service community who have also been trained in emergency stress and the debriefing process. They are not mental health professionals, but working providers who simply want to help their brother and sister rescuers in times of need.

The debriefing session is most commonly held a couple of days after the event. Often it takes a little while for the immediate shock of the incident to subside and for any stress reactions to take hold. During the initial 24 hours following a crisis, rescuers should be told about the possible stress reactions they can expect, be given simple stress defense techniques, and asked to report to the debriefing.

The Debriefing Session

1. **Introduction.** The debriefing team leader opens the session by emphasizing the importance of talking about feelings and reactions to an event as a way to heal and move on. He explains that powerful emotions may be unleashed by this process. Anger, frustration, guilt, sorrow and tears are all normal reactions to a critical incident. He points out that no notes will be taken, that everything that is said or experienced in the session, without exception, will be absolutely confidential, not to be discussed in any form with anyone not in the room.

2. **Facts.** Participants state their name and years of
   service. Then they describe what they did during the
   incident. This phase of the debriefing is neutral, a
   safe way to begin speaking of the powerful event.
   Rescuers aren't being asked to touch on their
   emotions, simply discuss the facts.
   Sometimes a participant does not want to go any farther than sharing the facts. The emotions are too
   frightening to take the process any deeper. But even
   these persons benefit from becoming aware of the
   thoughts and feelings of others, knowing they are
   not alone in their feelings.

3. **Thoughts.** The team leader may next ask, "*When you
   arrived on the scene and saw the condition of the victims
   involved, what did you think? What went through your mind as
   you proceeded to treat people? What did you think
   afterward?*"

   Now the event becomes more personal. The
   participants begin to consider how it affected them.
   The detachment that they may have maintained since
   the incident begins to fade. They start to
   consider the reality of what happened, to consider
   its actual impact.

   Not everyone will want to talk about their thoughts
   at this point. That's OK. Each person in the group
   must be comfortable with the process. Not everyone
   will be ready to move to a given level at the same
   time. Some, again, will never go any deeper. The
   leader will encourage people to talk, but never place
   anyone on the hot seat.

4. **Reactions.** This is the deepest stage of the process,
   where feelings about the event are accessed directly.
   The denial of emotion is one of the main causes of
   later stress reactions. Now participants are encour-
   aged to recognize that they are human, that they are
   subject to a wide range of emotions. Often the emotions conflict—sorrow mingles with anger or guilt.

The message here is: **It's OK not to be OK.**
Participants are asked to describe the one thing
that bothers them most about the event. It's an
opportunity to talk about all the feelings they've
been holding in. It allows them to bring it up, get
it out, and move on.

5. **Symptoms.** Participants next describe the way the
event has affected them in terms of objective signs and
symptoms. What's been happening since the incident?
What's happening now? They might talk about difficulty
sleeping, flashbacks to the incident, feelings of intense
sadness, crying spells, irritability, or any of the other
normal symptoms of intense stress.

    This phase helps the rescuers to move away from
their intense feelings and back to a more objective
view of things. It lets them know that the symptoms
they are experiencing are normal reactions, that
others are going through the same things.

6. **Teaching.** Next, the leader and counselors discuss
the reasons that symptoms arise, the mechanisms
of stress reaction, and the techniques for coping with
stress. Participants learn how to interact with their
families, what to say to them and how to say it.
Information is provided about the grief process if
appropriate.

    One of the most important things that
participants take away from a session is a mental
structure that allows them to make sense of the
strong and sometimes confusing thoughts and
emotions that an incident can generate. Knowledge
helps make stress more manageable.

    The teaching here is not formal instruction about
stress. It's simply a reinforcement of the idea that
what may be happening is normal, that the bad or
frightening feelings a rescuer may be experiencing are
to be expected. Often participants teach each other by
sharing their experiences.

7. **Re-entry.** In conclusion, the group is given an opportunity to sum up their experiences or to ask any remaining questions. Procedures for obtaining additional counseling and assistance are clearly outlined. Before the meeting winds down, the team leader again emphasizes the importance of confidentiality.

Awareness—

The more you put into CISD, the more benefit you get. Take some time to step back and look closely at what you've been through.

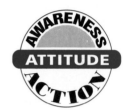

Attitude—

"It often takes more strength and courage to acknowledge and express emotions than it does to bottle them up. To seek help is a sign of strength, not weakness."

Action—

Attend the CISD session with an open mind. Make contact with the team leader or one of the peer counselors if you feel you need to talk more about the incident or could benefit from additional help. That's what they're there for.

Peer Support

Not every bad call will require the assistance of a debriefing team. But keep in mind that almost any serious incident can be critical for a given individual. Much more common than the disasters requiring formal CISD are the auto accidents or CPR calls that affect a single rescuer. In those cases, peer support can be crucial in dealing with the stress.

> *Peer counselors are able to provide a safe place for distressed emergency workers to get in touch with their feelings in a nonjudgemental environment.*

peer support The process by which one emergency responder helps another to deal with stress or with related problems.

The most important quality of a peer support person is a desire to assist a brother or sister rescuer in distress. It's not easy to take on another person's pain. You really have to be motivated to give assistance. The goal is to help the person talk freely about what has occurred. The process creates a beneficial release of emotion similar to what happens in a CISD session.

One EMT learned a lot about peer support from her 8-year-old daughter. *"Mary was feeling very sorry for the mother of her friend who had died after being struck by a car. One afternoon she decided to go over and visit her friend's mom. When she returned, I asked her what she had done to provide some comfort. Mary replied, 'I just sat in her lap and cried with her.'"*

This child summed up a lot of what peer support is about. It mainly means making yourself available, listening to the other person or just being with them and sharing their emotions.

What's a Friend For?

Peer support, in the final analysis, means being a friend. It actually starts with the little things. After any stressful call it's helpful to say to a colleague, *"You did a great job out there."* Or, *"Thanks for being there."* Or, *"That was a tough one, you really came through."* We all know how these few words can make a big difference in the way we feel about an event. None of us receives enough praise or thanks for what we do.

Empathy is another important quality in a peer support person. Empathy does not mean taking on the other person's emotion. It means appreciating what they are feeling, being able to see the situation from their point of view, understanding what's behind the opinions and feelings they are expressing. You understand the person who's having a problem with a bad call because you can imagine yourself in exactly the same situation.

Attitudes to Avoid During Peer Support

Authoritarian:
"Pull yourself together. Breaking down like this is just a cop out."

Blaming:
"If you'd followed the protocols, that guy would still be alive."

Moral:
"The rest of us are doing our jobs, what's the matter with you?"

Clinical:
"You're sick. You've really got problems."

Dismissive:
"Just forget about it. The call wasn't that bad."

Six Steps to Effective Peer Support

1. **Find out about the incident.** You should learn not only the general facts about the critical event, but details about what the individual rescuer did and saw during it. This will make it easier to understand why the person is upset.

2. **Never make judgments.** Accept the response that the person is having. Don't try to decide whether it's appropriate. The rescuer may be feeling anger, sadness, confusion, frustration, or guilt. Accept it, whatever it is. Suspend all judgment and criticism.

   At times you may feel it's appropriate to offer advice. The person may profit from your experiences as a peer. Share the things that worked for you after a difficult call. But remember that your main function is just to be supportive. Acknowledge that the person must find his or her own way to handle the incident.

3. **Listen to what the person is saying.** You have to pay attention to what they are telling you. Being there and holding the person's hand is important. But they also have to know that you are interested in what they are going through. Acknowledge the things they tell you and ask appropriate questions.

4. **Encourage communication.** Understand that the person may be reluctant to talk about something that is painful, or maybe embarrassing. Encourage them with comments like:

   "Tell me more about that."

   "This must have been a difficult experience for you."

   "Can you tell me what you were thinking?"

   "Have you experienced anything like this before?"

   "Tell me what you mean."

   "What was it like for you?"

   Nonverbal actions are another way to encourage communication and show your support. Sit down facing the person. Maintain eye contact. If you are comfortable doing so, touch the person—a hand on the shoulder or back can be a source of comfort at a time of isolation.

Alcohol should be avoided in these situations. While it can loosen inhibitions and stimulate talk, it tends to counteract the benefits of discussing the event. Afterward, the person feels "it was the alcohol talking." Drinking is rarely helpful in handling stress.

5. **Validate emotions.** One of the most common concerns after an incident is: Is it OK to feel this way? You are there to tell the person that it is OK, that the way they are feeling is normal and understandable, that it's OK not to be OK. For example, if they are feeling angry, you might acknowledge the feeling by saying, "*I can see how angry you are.*"

   Crying is often a part of the process. When emotions run high, tears flow. Crying provides a wonderful healing release and serves as an antidote to stress. Never try to stop the person from venting their emotions in tears. Pass the tissues and encourage them to weep as much as they feel like.

6. **Know your limits.** Realize that you are not a mental health professional. Whenever you have a sense that the person is not on the road to resolving the situation in a healthy way, it's time to recommend professional assistance. Some of the signs might be an inability to regain emotional control, prolonged sleeplessness or loss of appetite, extreme agitation, any talk of suicide or violence, any serious alcohol or drug abuse.

   Be on the lookout, too, for when you are becoming overloaded with the stress of offering support. Peer support is not an easy task. Don't let it overwhelm you. Find out about the CISD programs that are offered in your area. If one does not exist, learn where distressed emergency workers can go for help.

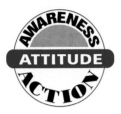

Awareness—

The people you work with might need peer support after any serious call. Be on the lookout for any signs that someone is not coping with the stress.

Attitude—

"My role is to be there for that person, to listen, to validate, not to judge."

Action—

Take the initiative in offering support, but don't intrude or force yourself on the person. Find a comfortable place to talk where you won't be disturbed. Start the conversation by just talking about what happened on the call.

For More Information

The International Critical Incident Stress Foundation assists in the development of CISD teams and disseminates stress-related information through its newsletter and other publications. They also run a 24-hour emergency hot line staffed by fire and police communications personnel. You can contact the Foundation at:

International Critical Incident Stress Foundation, Inc.
5018 Dorsey Hall Road - Suite 104
Ellicott City, MD 21042
410-730-4311 (Fax: 410-730-4313)
HOTLINE: 410-313-2473

(See also Resource Appendix)

SUMMARY

- A critical incident is any serious event that creates overwhelming stress in a emergency responder.
- Certain factors can contribute to turning a routine call into a critical incident. They include:

  Incidents involving children

  Trapped victims

  Line-of-duty deaths

  An incident involving a relative or close friend

  Violence

  Distraught bystanders

  Media attention

- No matter how experienced you are, no matter how many bad calls you've been through, it's always possible that the next call could be the "big one" for you.
- The stress that results from critical incidents is a normal reaction to an extraordinary event.
- Critical incident stress can combine with cumulative day-to-day stress to overwhelm a person when they don't expect it.
- It's important after a critical incident to be on the lookout for signs and symptoms that you are not handling the stress.
- Critical incident stress debriefing (CISD) is an effective way to prevent delayed stress reactions.
- The CISD session guides participants from cognitive areas to emotional areas and back again through seven steps:
    1. Introduction   5. Symptoms
    2. Facts   6. Teaching
    3. Thoughts   7. Re-entry
    4. Reactions
- During a critical incident some rescuers may suffer the effects of stress on the scene.

- Peer support plays an important part in the of stress reactions to critical incidents.
- A good peer support person listens well, encourages communication, withholds judgment, validates emotions, and when needed helps the rescuer to get professional counseling.

For Further Thought

1. Think about certain calls that have bothered you more than others even though the incident may not have involved a crisis. What were the factors that made it more difficult for you? How did others react?

2. Why is it that no one, no matter how much experience they may have, is immune to the effects of a bad call?

3. A famous statement goes, *"All we have to fear is fear itself."* How might this apply to critical incident stress?

4. Why might it be important that even those who feel they have no need for stress debriefing attend a CISD session when it is offered after a disaster?

5. Since the goal of a debriefing is to talk about feelings, why not start out with a discussion of what each person felt at the scene?

6. Discuss some ways you might initiate peer support with a colleague who has been through one of these events:
   - Treated patients at a multi-casualty motor vehicle accident.
   - Been on an unsuccessful CPR call for a 45-year-old male who suffered a heart attack.
   - Responded to a drowning involving a 10-year-old boy.
   - Had to deal with a mother who saw her son struck by a car and killed.

7. After a critical incident rescuers often feel that the powerful emotions they feel are indications of weakness or mental illness. What are some ways to validate these emotions so that they don't snowball into even greater stress?

CHAPTER 7

Stress Defense

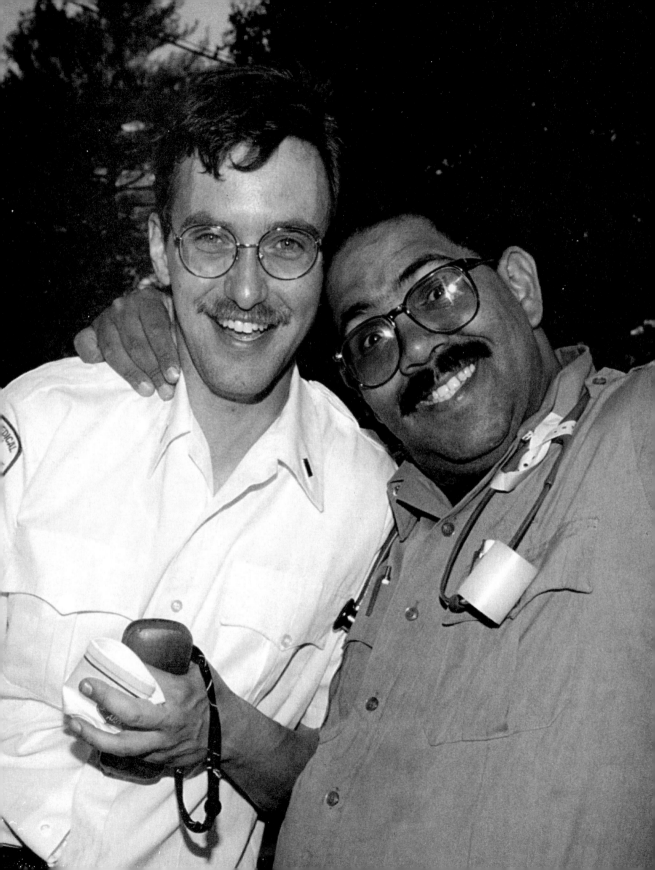

Stress Defense

Remember the story of the saber-toothed tiger? In the face of danger, your body gears up to give you a better chance to confront the menace or to get away from it—the fight or flight reaction. But when you experience that arousal today, the stimulus is often something you can't fight and can't run away from. You're left with the arousal and no way to release it in physical action. The effect of that pent up energy on your mind and body is stress.

Learning to Flow

Stress is a fact of life, and it is something you have to deal with throughout your life. This is particularly true for the emergency worker. While you sometimes release a portion of your fight or flight arousal in the physical activity of a call, often a great deal of it is left over afterward. It adds up. The additional stress that everyone experiences on the job and in daily life also contributes to cumulative stress. What happens? You're all charged up with nowhere to go. The way to defend yourself against the effects of stress is to learn to flow.

The whole concept of stress defense is summed up in two rules.

Rule #1: Don't sweat the small stuff.

Life is full of small stuff. The problem is, we often blow it out of proportion. We turn a small event into a major crisis. We experience the arousal and the stress that goes along with it. Because we believe it's big, we react as if it were.

Rule #2: It's all small stuff.

Think about it. The definition of "big stuff" is something you can't recover from. In the final analysis, that means death—your death. Events may drastically and permanently change the quality of your life. You will certainly experience losses and setbacks. But if you're alive you can recover or adapt and move on. You're still in the flow of life.

VIII Don't Sweat the Small Stuff

To let go of regrets and remorse and worries is not a cop out. It doesn't mean you don't feel or grieve. It means you recognize that life is a flow, that regretting what you can't change or fretting about what might happen next week is a waste of time and energy.

"The key to happiness," the saying goes, "is not to get what you want—but to want what you get."

"The key to happiness," the saying goes, "is not to get what you want—but to want what you get."

To flow means to recognize that you have all the resources you need to cope with whatever situation arises. The idea of flow is the idea of practical optimism. You can handle the issues that face you. There are opportunities out there. Difficulties will be resolved. Things really could be worse. So you keep it in perspective and move on.

A famous prayer asks for "the courage to change what I can change and the serenity to accept what I can't change—and the wisdom to know the difference." That sums up the idea of flow.

Tools for Stress Defense

"I bought my 6-year-old a globe when she started first grade," a volunteer EMT said. "One night I'd been out on two calls, it was three in the morning, I had problems at work to face the next day, and I was feeling stressed. I happened to glance at the globe on the shelf. I saw where my town, my state was. And I noticed what a

large world there was out there. Just that bit of perspective seemed to take a weight off my shoulders. It gave me a little lift, and I was able to go back to sleep peacefully."

Don't sweat the small stuff. Sometimes something as simple as a globe can remind you to flow rather than to fight. The stress defenses in this chapter will help you to counteract the negative effects of stress in your life. They are the tools of wellness as much as of stress management. They help you to move in a positive direction, toward flowing, relaxing, and renewing.

These defenses are useful for dealing with stress when it builds, when you start to experience the signs and symptoms of the cumulative tensions in your life. But they're even more useful for prevention. Every emergency responder should choose the tools that work best and make them a habit before stress builds.

stress defense
Any regular action you take to prevent the stress of daily life from accumulating.

Awareness—

Be alert to your own signs that stress is building. When you detect any of them—sleeplessness, irritability, headaches—getting back into the flow becomes a necessity.

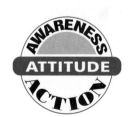

Attitude—

"I'm going to treat myself the way I would like others to treat me. I can and will make the adjustments in my lifestyle that will keep me healthy and help me to cope with stress."

Action—

You need to practice in order to use any tool. Even relaxation requires practice. Act to turn the stress defense tools into habits. Begin today. Find the stress defenses that are suited to you.

Secrets of Relaxation

To try to relax is a contradiction in terms. To relax means to stop trying. It seems easy, but it can often be the hardest thing in the world.

Relaxation is a skill. It requires practice. There are many tools that can help you to relax, from music to exercise, simple daydreaming, meditation, or an involving hobby. The important thing is to find some tool that works for you and to use it regularly.

Building strength in muscles requires you to alternately work and relax them. A state of constant tension only leads to fatigue. Always being busy and tense leads to burnout. To stay healthy requires you to relax regularly.

Three Rules of Relaxation

1. **Give yourself permission to relax**. Achievement-oriented emergency responders often have trouble taking this step. There's always one more piece of business to take care of. Relaxation seems like a luxury. It's not. It's a necessary part of keeping yourself well.

2. **Create a peaceful space.** Find a place where you won't be disturbed. It should be quiet, away from the distractions that normally grab your attention. It could be a bedroom, a study, or a patio. It might be your basement or garage. Assume a comfortable position.

3. **Use a mental device.** Don't just sit there waiting to relax. You need to occupy your mind. Music is often helpful. Reading a book or magazine can be relaxing, but don't choose something related to EMS.

The One-Minute Vacation

All the events of your life are recorded in your mind, along with the emotions that accompanied them. When you recall a tense incident from the past, you feel some of that tension. When you bring to mind a pleasant experience, some of the feeling of relaxation and enjoyment comes with it. Imagery can help you to gain a few minutes of peace when you need it. The one-minute vacation is a practice in imagery. All it requires is for you to recall a wonderful time in your life, maybe a vacation, a memorable holiday. The important point is to use an image from reality, not a fantasy.

Begin by thinking of a pleasant vacation you've had. It might have been at the lake, in the mountains, a camping trip, or an excursion to Disney World.

Relive the vacation as clearly as you can. Take out your photo album or look at the video you shot. Imagine yourself back there, smelling the air, listening to the sound of the ocean, experiencing the fun of it.

Select one photo that sums up the experience for you. Hold it in your hand, look at it, imprint the image in your mind. Close your eyes and experience the scene the photo brings back. Look at the picture again, close your eyes and live the scene again. Do this a few more times.

This image becomes a tool for your one-minute vacation. The next time you are feeling stressed, take a minute to step back. Take a deep breath and tell yourself to relax, to let go. Do it again. Now close your eyes and recall the image you imprinted. Use as many senses as you can to relive the experience, the sights, sounds, smells.

After a minute, take another deep breath, hold it for 3 to 5 seconds, and exhale through your mouth, telling yourself to relax and let go. Open your eyes and return to your activity.

The one-minute vacation will give you some of the benefits of a real vacation. Imagery is a powerful tool. When you allow yourself to picture the vacation in your mind, you will be transported briefly to a time of peace and happiness.

Also, since you can only hold one thought in your mind at a time, the positive thoughts will replace any negative thoughts you may be experiencing. This will help you to stay in control and avoid giving in to stress. Try it, trust in the process. It does work.

The Calming Phrase

An even quicker way to gain control during stressful situations is to use a calming phrase. The phrase, when stated aloud or to yourself, can bring thoughts of peace to your mind.

As with the one-minute vacation, the phrase will be based on an experience in your life. It can represent any event or idea that you find particularly calming.

One Advanced EMT talked about the phrase he uses in stressful situations:

"I found that whenever I was confronted with a stressful situation I would begin to act in a negative way. My heart would pound, I'd feel anxious. When stress was really powerful I had trouble making decisions. This really bothered me on calls.

"When I first heard the idea of the calming phrase described, I thought it was a stupid thing to do. I couldn't see that just saying something would calm me down. But I needed help, so I gave it a try.

"The phrase I use is: 'Wait a minute—is this any way for a gentle, flowing mountain stream to respond?'"

He explained that the image evoked a cabin in the mountains where he'd once gone on vacation. Across the road was a stream called Betty Brook. It wound through pine trees and bubbled over rocks. It was a peaceful place where time seemed to stand still.

"My buddies think I'm nuts, but whenever I need to regain control of a stressful situation, I repeat my calming phrase. I remember the night of the plane crash. Throughout the rescue,

whenever I felt myself reacting to the stress, I would say the phrase. Each time, I would be transported briefly back to Betty Brook. I would regain control and be able to go on with what I had to do."

It's a simple technique, but it works.

Breathe to Relax

How can you quickly regain control in a stressful situation? How can you bring physical and emotional reactions under control when you are in the midst of a crisis? The simple answer is: **Breathe.**

Everyone involved in emergency medicine has the ABCs drilled into them. Airway and breathing top the list when you assess any patient. Just as breathing is important for maintaining life, it can be a powerful regulator of your reaction to stress.

Often, your reaction to a crisis is to hold your breath. You do it without thinking. You breathe in shallow gulps, just using the tops of your lungs.

But if you turn your attention to your breathing, force yourself to take slow, deep breaths, you physically counteract the effects of the stress. You'll find the tension easing a bit, a feeling of control coming back.

Here's an exercise that is useful any time stress strikes:

- Become aware of your breathing.
- Begin with a long, deep inhalation. Allow your lungs to fill from bottom to top.
- Hold the breath for 3 to 5 seconds.
- Forcefully exhale through your mouth, telling yourself to relax and let go.

Repeat the process once or twice.

Another way to use your breathing as a stress defense is to take an *oxygen break* instead of a coffee break. You don't need pure oxygen to do it. All that's required is a series of long, deep breaths. If you can, step outside. Breathe in and out through your nose. Expand your lungs fully, then let the breath flow out at its own rate. Do this 10 times. You'll find that it helps clear your head, energize you and relax you at the same time.

Stress Barriers

A career paramedic said:

"My wife and I always seemed to get into some kind of argument the minute I walked in the door at night. I would be beat from the tour and the drive home. I needed some time to unwind before I got into any serious conversation or began to play with the kids. It seemed like we were fighting all the time. We ended up at a marriage counselor.

"The therapist asked me what I needed. I said, 'I need some space when I get home.' He asked, 'How could you get this space?' I thought about it and said, 'Maybe if I took a nice, long hot shower.' My wife agreed to give me this space, and I agreed to do some of the things that were important to her.

"I began to take a shower when I first got home. I found that it really allowed me to unwind. I would stand in the hot water, let my muscles go, think about a relaxing idea. My hot water bill may be higher, but my stress is lower."

> **A stress barrier is anything that separates you from the stress of daily life, the tension created by your job or your EMS work.**

A stress barrier is anything that separates you from the stress of daily life, the tension created by your job or your EMS work. It can be a shower, a peaceful walk, a jog or other light exercise, even a cup of hot chocolate. It's something you do that blocks the worries and stresses of one part of your life from seeping into other parts.

Winding Down After a Call

"My problem," one EMT said, "is trying to relax after a call. It seems like once the adrenaline gets into my system I stay keyed up for hours. It's especially bad at night. Even if I go out on a routine call, I just can't get back to sleep when I return home. Sometimes I lie in bed the rest of the night staring at the ceiling."

Almost everyone involved in EMS experiences this problem at times. The first rule is about what not to do. Don't finish up a call with a cigarette, a cup of coffee, or a can of soda. Don't use alcohol to unwind.

Instead, develop a routine that gives you an opportunity to let off some of the tension that's built up. A glass of water is the best refreshment. If you're going back to bed, the calcium in a glass of milk can help you to relax. A short walk is ideal. The breathing exercises described earlier will help. You can combine the two, breathing deeply as you walk. Use some mental imagery. After a call is a good time for a one-minute vacation.

Some emergency responders find that it's helpful to write down the details of the call. Note in particular any issue that remains unresolved—something you might have done differently, a conflict with a colleague. And write how you felt at different points during the call. This can help you to avoid repeatedly going over the events in your mind.

Music can help you to relax after a call or at other times. A paramedic told how she learned to use music to unwind:

"I listen to my Walkman a lot," she said. "I used to always put on rock music. A friend lent me an environmental tape that combines the sounds of nature with classical music. It was so soothing I bought the tape for myself.

"One day at work we had a very bad call, a kid hit by a train. Back at the station I put on my 'Solitudes' tape. As I listened to this peaceful music, I could feel my mind and body quieting. Now I always use music as a way to unwind after stress."

The Seven Deadly Sins

Research involving 7,000 people in California found that the following habits correlate with illness and early death:

1. Excessive alcohol consumption
2. Smoking
3. Being overweight
4. Sleeping too little or too much
5. Not getting enough exercise
6. Eating between meals
7. Not eating breakfast

Exercise: Antidote to Stress

Exercise is one of the most important ways to keep the stresses in your life from overwhelming you. Stress is an arousal for action. Exercise releases much of the resulting tension. It leaves you relaxed and invigorated.

The key is to devise a regular program of exercise that fits your lifestyle and your needs. The object is not to turn yourself into an athlete, but to do enough to counteract the negative effects of stress and to maintain the well-being of your body.

We all have excuses. Too busy to exercise? You can achieve an acceptable level of fitness by exercising for as little as 30 minutes three times a week. Anyone can adjust their schedule to fit that in.

Too tired to exercise? You may be tired because you don't exercise. Exercise actually increases your store of energy and prepares you to cope with the challenges you meet in your daily life.

Take a minute to consider those challenges:

You are sound asleep in bed. The alarm sounds. You awaken with a start. Your heart pounds as you rush to dress, hurry to your car. Your heart rate is up to 120. At the scene you treat a patient who weighs 220 pounds. He needs to be carried up from a basement apartment. In the ambulance he goes into cardiac arrest. You perform CPR all the way to the hospital.

Is your body ready for this demand? Regular exercise is the only way to prepare.

> ## Before You Begin
>
> It's a good idea to see your doctor before you begin any regular exercise, and talk about what you'll be doing. Here are the recommended steps you should take if you're about to start on a new exercise program.
>
> - Under 30: You're OK if you've had a check-up in the past year and have no medical problems.
>
> - Age 30-39: Have a check-up within three months of beginning, including an electrocardiogram at rest.
>
> - Age 40-59: A check-up and a stress test within three months.
>
> - Over 59: A check-up and stress test immediately before you begin your program.
>
> Never try to undo years of inactivity by plunging into a program of heavy exercise. Easy does it.

You should be looking for three results from your exercise:

1. **Cardio-respiratory endurance.** This is the most important. It can be built up by walking, jogging, swimming, biking, or any other exercise that requires effort over time.

2. **Flexibility.** Bad backs are the bane of emergency service. Regular stretching keeps you limber and reduces your chances of injury.

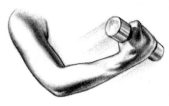

3. Muscular strength. Some strength is necessary to perform in your work. Exercising enough to maintain muscle tone contributes to overall fitness.

An ideal exercise regime will cover all three areas. Today almost everyone has access to fitness centers or formal exercise programs. Information about fitness is easy to obtain. Therefore no one has a legitimate excuse not to get some regular exercise.

Six Rules of Effective Exercise

1. **Warm up.** Before you begin your workout, warm your muscles with light exercise. Always start slow and build up in intensity.

2. **Avoid pain.** "No pain, no gain" should never be your motto. In fact, experts warn that pain is a sign that you are exercising improperly.

3. **Stretch afterward.** It's essential to stretch after your workout. Stretching will minimize sore or stiff muscles later.

4. **Regularity is the key.** Light exercise every day is the best approach to fitness. Don't try to be a "weekend athlete," working out hard once or twice a week.

5. **Make it fun.** The best exercise is the exercise you enjoy. Consider softball, golf, swimming, tennis, whatever activity gives you pleasure.

6. **Take advantage of hidden exercise.** Walk up a couple of flights of stairs instead of taking the elevator. Get off the bus two blocks before your stop. Gardening, raking leaves, dancing, all of these activities have been shown to improve fitness and can be effective stress defenses in themselves.

Walking for Fitness

Walking is the ideal exercise. It's easy. It requires no equipment or preparation. You can always fit it into your schedule. It relaxes you while it tones your muscles and gives your cardiovascular system a workout. Recent studies have shown that walking is almost as beneficial as running when it comes to fitness.

Walking can become the foundation of your exercise program. All you need to do is to find a way to regularly incorporate it into your day. Walk to work. Or park a few blocks from where you work and walk the rest of the way. Walk when you get home from work. Walk in the park. If the weather's bad, take a couple of laps around your local mall. Walk upstairs instead of using the elevator.

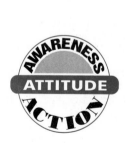

One excellent stress defense is to walk with a friend or your spouse. A regular walk is a great way to gain time to talk and to participate together in an uncomplicated activity. Make it a habit.

One busy paramedic had this advice: *"When I used to go to the mall I would fight the traffic trying to park as close to the entrance as I could. Now I do just the opposite. I park as far away as I can. I get some exercise and avoid most of the hassles of parking."*

Awareness—

A completely sedentary life can contribute to the effects of stress. When we're busy we can slide out of the habit of regular exercise. Keep track of the number of times you exercise in a week. How do you feel after you've exercised?

Attitude—

"I don't need to be an athlete in order to exercise. I can easily fit a program of regular activity into my life."

Action—

Shape your program to you—your level of fitness, your needs, your schedule. Build up gradually. Regularity is much more important than intensity.

Eat Right to Stay Healthy

"I was working steady midnight shifts," one career EMT said. "I would come home in the morning too tired to eat. I would wake up late in the afternoon not wanting dinner, but not really wanting breakfast either. I would just eat what was around.

"By the time I would leave for work at 2230 hours, I'd be hungry. On my way to the station house I would stop at Dunkin Donuts, get my large coffee and two of my favorite donuts. This is the food that started my tour. Usually around three in the morning we would order bacon and egg sandwiches from the diner. This became my habit of eating day after day. If it wasn't eggs, it was cheeseburgers deluxe. I gained 35 pounds, weighed more than I ever had in my life. I had to be fitted for a new uniform. At my annual medical my cholesterol level was 398. That did it. I had to do something."

The 80/20 Rule of Eating Well

This rule states that you should be certain that 80 percent of your diet is healthy: fruit, vegetables, grain, lean meat. Then you can stop worrying about the other 20 percent, which can consist of pizza, milkshakes, and rich desserts.

Too many emergency responders are, like this man, burning the nutrition candle at both ends. On the one hand, stress can adversely affect eating habits. Often the person who's anxious reaches for food as a consolation. A pressured feeling prompts a person to grab a burger and fries rather than take time to eat a balanced meal.

The excess weight that comes from poor eating habits puts further strain on the body and the mind.

On the other hand, stress drains the body of key vitamins and minerals and makes it even more vital for us to eat a well-rounded diet in order to maintain wellness. Calcium and vitamin C in particular are affected by stress. Stress reactions stimulate the adrenal glands to produce the adrenaline that puts you into overdrive. Adrenaline depletes the body of vitamin C. Since vitamin C plays an important role in maintaining the immune system, a lack of it can lead to frequent illnesses. The EMT was out sick so often he was labeled a "sick leave abuser."

Calcium absorption is also affected by stress. Calcium plays a role in keeping your heartbeat steady and regulating the nervous system. B vitamins are important for allowing your body to respond properly to stress. These elements must be replenished daily.

The best way to make sure you are getting proper nutrition is to eat a balanced diet, with an emphasis on grains, vegetables, and fruit. Vitamin supplements are not an antidote to a poor diet.

Moderation: The Key to Healthy Eating

If your eating habits are actually contributing to the ill effects of stress you can easily turn the situation around without drastic diets. The first step is to begin to eat *"heart smart."* Cut down on fats and sweets, load up on complex carbohydrates like pasta, vegetables, and whole-grain bread. Substitute fish or chicken for red meat. Limit fried foods. Watch the snacks.

Moderation doesn't mean you can never enjoy a steak or a pizza. It just means that if you're going to eat a T-bone tonight, don't load up on sausages and eggs at breakfast. Have a salad for lunch, then enjoy your big meal in the evening.

Here are some aspects of nutrition that emergency responders need to be especially aware of:

Caffeine. Taken in excess, it's a significant contributor to stress. If you're drinking more than a couple of cups of coffee a day, you're not doing yourself any good. Tea and soft drinks often contain caffeine too. It's important to consider your total intake of caffeine, which may be higher than you think.

"Consolation eating." You eat not because you're hungry but because you feel stressed. It's a habit to avoid whenever possible.

Sugar. Donuts and candy are not a good way to boost your energy level. In fact they tend to quickly deplete your blood sugar and leave you drained. Keep in mind that the average 12-ounce soft drink contains 11 teaspoons of pure sugar.

Breakfast. Don't skip it. You need the nourishment of a good breakfast. Make it a nutritious meal. Add fruit, yogurt, whole-wheat bread, cereal. It can make a big difference.

The "quick fix." Donuts and coffee, a bacon and egg sandwich, a pepperoni pizza—avoid the temptation to beat your hunger to death rather than satisfy it. With a little planning it takes no more time to eat a healthy, stress-free diet.

Eating on the run. Working in emergency service often makes scheduling meals difficult. You grab whatever is available. To solve the problem, get in the habit of bringing your lunch or dinner with you. At least have a nutritious snack available to hold you over.

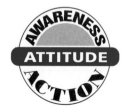

Awareness—

Am I paying attention to what I'm eating? Have I gotten into eating habits that are contributing to my stress, causing me to gain weight, sapping my energy?

Attitude—

"I don't need junk food, coffee, sweets or soft drinks. If I eat them occasionally I balance out my diet with nutritious foods at other times."

Action—

You need to plan a stress-defense diet. It starts in the supermarket—buy plenty of healthy foods. If you snack, make sure you have foods on hand that aren't loaded with sugar and salt. For a while you might want to keep track of what you eat to assure that you're getting enough fruits, vegetables and carbohydrates.

An Active Mind

A mind, the saying goes, is a terrible thing to waste. You already understand the important role of the mind in regulating your reaction to stress.

One paramedic talked about his decision to earn his pilot's license:

"I always wanted to do it, never had time. Something always got in the way. Finally I made myself try it. It's been the most exciting challenge in my life in a long time. It made me use my head again. It feels good. I actually think this adventure has made me sharper on the ambulance. It's like I've learned to think again."

Your mind needs exercise and stimulation just as your body does. Broad interests, and an alert and active mind are crucial defenses against stress.

What you want to avoid are long periods of passive entertainment. One firefighter discussed how he would come home from his shift, crash on the couch, and stare at the TV for hours. He said, *"Most of the time I didn't even know what was on. It was just white noise, helping me to escape."*

Better to follow the example of the person who put his energy into learning to fly. There are many activities that absorb and stimulate your mind. Take a formal course, learn on your own, or simply pursue a favorite hobby. Take up photography. Learn to play a musical instrument—it's never too late to try. Take a cooking course. Read history books or biographies. Learn to paint. Plant a garden.

One way to find an absorbing activity is to return to an interest you had as a child. Maybe you took piano lessons but then gave it up. Maybe you always liked to draw, or to fix engines, or to collect coins. Many people find great pleasure in renewing these old interests.

Look on the Light Side

Emergency service is a serious business. When people call upon you, it's not to come and have a good time with

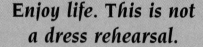

Enjoy life. This is not a dress rehearsal.

them. They call when they are sick, injured, or dying. It's a grim world you see out there. If you're not careful the negativity can seep into your life and add to your stress. To survive you need to cultivate a positive attitude and use humor as an energizer.

You already know that humor can be very useful in EMS. It helps to ease patients' fears and build rapport with them. It relieves the tension of a bad call. It counteracts the stressful events that you encounter every day.

IX   Take Time To Laugh

Laughter has been described as "internal jogging." A good laugh increases positive emotions, boosts self-esteem, and clears your mind.

Here are some simple suggestions for using humor as a stress defense:

- **Build a file of jokes and cartoons.** Save anything that strikes you as funny. Use them when you need a humor lift. This is also a useful device for those who can never remember a joke.

- **Take the time to send a funny card or joke to a friend.** Sharing humor is the best way to enjoy it—it gives both of you a lift.

- **See a funny movie or rent a video.** Go with friends. Break the cycle of serious life.

- **Look for the humor in life.** It's always there. You just have to be willing to find it.

- **Learn to laugh at yourself.** It's the best way to put your problems in perspective.

A Note About Black Humor

People who work in emergency service joke about death. They joke about serious illness. They joke about tragic events. Everyone who's worked in EMS has heard this type of black humor. It often comes out after an especially bad call or a difficult day. Usually it's not really very funny, but it serves as a short-term release for the powerful emotions that are otherwise held inside. Someone's laughing to keep from crying.

Black humor will always be a part of EMS work. But keep two points in mind:

- At a certain point, black humor becomes a sign of excess stress. If you feel so removed from humane feelings for your patients that everything to you is a joke, you need to take a very close look at how you are dealing with the pressures of EMS work.

- Imagine walking out of the ER and making a crude joke about the critically ill patient you've just left off—

then turning to find the patient's spouse standing there listening. Even the possibility of that happening should make you hesitate before using any black humor. Remember, you're a professional. Act like one.

Getting Away From It All

Modern life tends to put everyone in a cocoon. Your home becomes the mother cocoon. Your car is a mobile cocoon that takes you to your job and the other places you habitually visit—satellite cocoons. Your life becomes severely restricted. You don't even go out to the movies, you simply drive your mobile cocoon to the video store and come back to hibernate in the mother cocoon. Life becomes a routine. You never break out of your environment.

Living your life in a rut is just the opposite of what you need. Variety and stimulation are important ways to keep stress from building up.

One seasoned firefighter told a group of younger members that they should plan to get out of town periodically.

"The town survived before you joined the department. It will survive if you go away for a weekend or a day. You cannot do this work all the time. You can't be ready to respond without taking a break occasionally. You need time for you and your family. Get out of town. When you come back your batteries will be charged and you'll be ready to roll."

Make Your Vacation Pay

A vacation is an excellent antidote to stress. To get the best results:

- Take at least two weeks off. A few days now and then isn't long enough to break your routine.
- Don't do the same thing every year.
- Don't take work with you.
- Get as far away from your usual life as you can.

The 24/365 Syndrome

What this veteran was talking about was the idea that you have to be ready to respond around the clock, every day of the year. You always have your pager with you. Always, in the back of your mind, you're "on," you're ready to drop what you're doing and respond to an emergency.

The **24/365 Syndrome** aggravates the stress that you're already feeling. It prevents you from ever really stepping back from your emergency duties. You never quite relax completely. A part of you is always in an emergency mode. This syndrome can be especially serious for those who work in EMS as a profession and then volunteer with their community rescue squad as well.

There's a life beyond the job—find it.

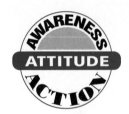

Awareness—

When was the last time I was completely away from my emergency service duties?

Attitude—

"The world will go on fine without me responding to every possible call. It's more important to keep my life in balance."

Action—

Turn off your pager. It's as simple as that. Do it for a day, an afternoon, an hour. And do it regularly.

Using Your Free Time

Free time can be an important stress defense if you use it wisely. This requires the three P's: **Plan, Positive, and Playful.**

It's crucial to *plan* stress-reducing activities. It may sound contradictory to plan free time, but too often household chores, errands and trivia eat into our free time until it's gone.

Plan. Make an appointment with yourself. Block out a certain amount of time on a regular basis for planned free-time activities. Don't let other duties and demands interfere. Keep that appointment.

Positive. Do something you enjoy that makes you feel good about yourself.

Playful. Children, who naturally turn to play when they're let loose, have something to teach adults. Play is time out from stress. It's whatever you do just for the fun of it. If you're the golfer who swears at a slice or a tennis player prone to throwing your racket, look for another activity.

Here are some of the ways you can turn free time into a stress defense:

The day trip. Break out of your cocoon for a day. Take a drive to the ocean, a lake, the mountains, or a favorite park. Do anything that breaks up your routine and removes you from your usual environment.

A hobby. One firefighter/EMT talked about his hobby, model trains:

"I still play with trains. I've loved them since the first set my parents gave me when I was little. Today my trains are in my back yard. I've become involved in the hobby of 'Garden Railroading.' I have the fun of the gardens and trains combined.

"When I'm playing with my trains, the stress of the world dis-appears. It's time to recharge my batteries. I believe my play makes me more effective at what I do all day long. You've got to take time to play. Life's too serious—and too short—not to have fun."

A hobby can be anything: a ball team, bowling, garden-ing, cooking, photography, wood working.

A day of rest. Do your weekends tend to fill in with work? Meetings, drills, shopping, errands, a part-time job, studying for a course—it leaves little time to relax. But a day of real relaxation every week is an excellent antidote for stress. You need it. Choose a day and protect it from intrusions.

"My hour." Try to schedule an hour every day that's just for yourself. Take a walk, write in a journal, devote it to any activity that you can do alone. Keep in mind that solitude can serve as a useful time to relax and reflect.

Health days. We all know about sick days. Sometimes it's a good idea to take a "health day" off from work. When you feel the stress building, take a day off before you get sick. Use it for rest and relaxation. Think of it as preventive medicine.

Ten Tips For
Defending

1. Buy a package of red self-stick dots. Put them on any item in your environment that tends to be a source of stress for you: the telephone, the drawer where you keep your bills, the clock, your EMT textbook, whatever it is. The dot is a reminder to step back, take a breath, and sidestep stress.

2. Drop out for a day or two. Make yourself completely inaccessible. Change your habits.

3. Set aside some "worry time." As minor problems and irritations come up during the day, put off worrying about them until a set time. Use that time to go over your concerns and plan effective actions.

4. Get away from your workplace on your breaks if you can. A change of scene, even a walk around the parking lot, can help relieve stress.

5. Soak in a hot bath.

6. Use an answering machine to get away from the pressure of the telephone. Return the calls when *you* feel like it.

7. Spend some time alone.

Against Stress

8. Get a pet. A cat or dog, even tropical fish, can provide a relaxing diversion.

9. Take a day to be good to yourself. Fill it with your favorite activities. Indulge yourself.

10. To fight time pressures, always leave gaps in your schedule. An unscheduled half hour here and there will keep you from getting backed up, and can serve as a welcome break.

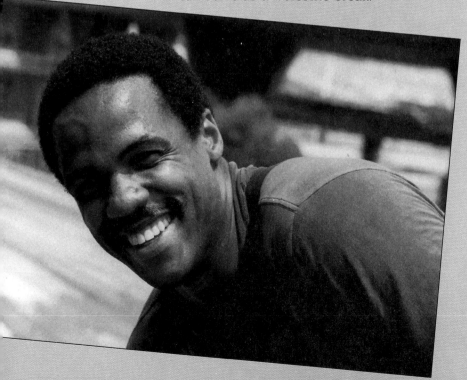

Your Social Support System

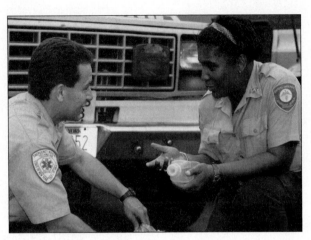

You might think of your friends as a stress safety net. They can alert you when you're just not handling the pressures of your life, and they can be there to support you when you need someone to talk to, or when you need to know you have people in your corner.

Without this support system, stress can make you feel very isolated. When you have no one to turn to or to talk to it's easy to lose perspective on the problems you face. It's easy to feel you're alone against the world.

While your spouse will obviously play an important role in your support system, it's not enough to depend solely on your husband or wife, or some other person to whom you're emotionally bound. Your social net must extend beyond your immediate family. Sometimes you'll need a sympathetic third party with whom you can talk about problems affecting your home life.

Your social supports must also extend beyond the people you know in EMS. Emergency work can create very deep friendships. But too many emergency responders limit their circle of friends to the rescue squad or fire department. You need more perspective. Make sure you socialize regularly with people who have no connection to the emergency service aspect of your life.

Make friends before you need them. When you are in need of assistance and support it's too late to go out and look for people to provide it. Remember that stress tends to push you into isolation.

The best strategy for building a support network is to be someone who gives to others. Let people know they can depend on you. *"A true friend,"* someone said, *"is the person who steps in when the world steps out."*

Talk It Over

When things build up, it helps to discuss your feelings. Talk with someone you trust and respect. Sometimes another person can help you see a different side to your problem.

Just as important is to be open to the help of others. If someone offers advice, listen to it carefully and let them know you appreciate it. Allow people to help you out when you're in need.

Awareness—

Regularly ask yourself:

- Who would I turn to in a time of powerful need?
- Do I have a network of friends that I spend time with off the job?
- Have I become isolated from most of the people I know?
- Who will be there for me when I feel most pressured?

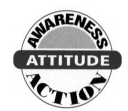

Attitude—

"I can widen my social support system by making specific efforts to do so. All it takes is a caring attitude and an offer of friendship."

Action—

Start by calling or visiting someone you haven't had contact with in a while. Friendships need to be maintained by keeping in touch.

Calm, Purpose and Adventure

All of the stress defenses we've discussed can help you to survive in the world of emergency response. They are even more useful when applied in the context of a purposeful life. Having clear goals and a definite direction in life is the best defense against stress.

A sense of purpose gives you an inner calm because it clarifies what you're doing and why. Even more important, it turns your life into an adventure. You may not achieve every goal you set your sights on, but you will come to see that the journey is the reward, that what's important is to try.

Set Goals to Give Your Life Purpose and Adventure

Usually you don't need to search for a purpose or to set new goals. What's really required is to sit down and *clarify* your life. What's important to you? Where do you want to be five years from now? What are your priorities? You'll find that you do have goals, but that you may not have made them specific before.

A periodic review of the direction your life is taking can be very useful. Look at it in terms of short-, medium-, and long-term goals. As you accomplish your short-term goals, set new ones, always with an eye on where you ultimately want to be.

Positive Addictions

Positive addictions are activities that become habits, but that benefit rather than damage you. A positive addiction should be an easy activity that you can do alone, that you can improve in over time, and that does not prompt you to criticize yourself.

Examples include biking, gardening, journal writing, music, swimming and meditating. It usually takes several months for the activity to become a real habit.

SUMMARY

- The two basic rules of stress defense are:
    1. Don't sweat the small stuff.
    2. It's all small stuff.
- Life goes on for those who choose to go on—if you can't fight and you can't flee, you need to flow.
- Prevention is the best way to defend yourself against stress.
- The three secrets of relaxation are:
    1. Give yourself permission to relax.
    2. Create a peaceful space.
    3. Use a mental device.
- A one-minute vacation is a way to take a step back from stress.
- A calming phrase is an even quicker method for getting yourself under control in a stressful situation.
- Deep breathing can help you to defend against stress during a crisis and relax you over the long run.
- Stress barriers are the relaxing activities that separate you from the stresses of work.
- Avoid coffee, soda, or alcohol when you return from an emergency.
- Exercise is a key stress defense.
- Walking is an ideal form of exercise.
- Those who are exposed to stress on a regular basis should pay close attention to what they eat.
- Humor is a necessary balance to the stressful situations you encounter in EMS work—take time to laugh.
- To avoid the **24/365 Syndrome** make sure you have a life away from EMS.

- Build a social support system before you need it.
- A sense of calm and the excitement of adventure both grow out of the purpose you set for your life.

For Further Thought

1. What are some things in EMS work that cause stress, but that we really can do nothing about? An example might be the drunk driver who causes an accident. What are some ways to flow with these things rather than let them contribute to stress?

2. We all have excuses about why we can't take time to relax. What are three of yours?

3. Talk about some specific ways for winding down after a call that leaves you tense.

4. Think of some ways you could fit exercise into your current lifestyle. For example, by riding a stationary bike while you watch the news on television.

5. How does your emergency service work contribute to poor eating habits (for example, the refrigerator full of soda and beer at the station house)? What are some ways to counteract those influences?

6. Is black humor something that we should avoid altogether? Does it serve a purpose? What are some reasons that EMS people use it?

7. Do you lack free time for yourself because you tend to give everything else a higher priority? What are some ways around this problem?

8. What are some specific things a person can do to build a social support network? Why are friends such an important stress defense?

CHAPTER 8

Stress and the Emergency Service Family

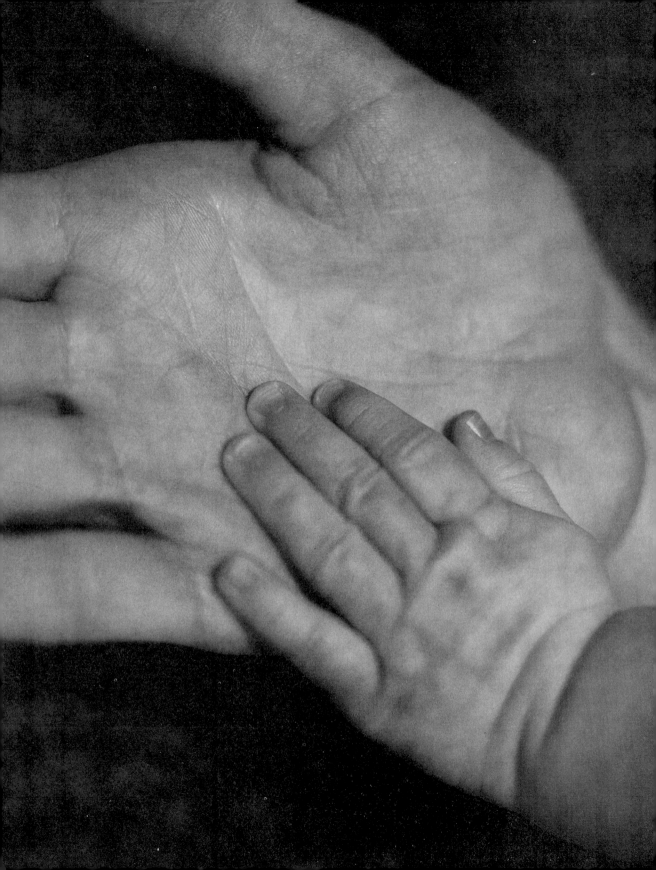

Stress and the Emergency Service Family

In addition to working as a career police officer, Steve was captain of his community rescue squad. He and his wife Pam had planned for several weeks to have a night out together.

"I was looking forward to the evening," Pam said. "Steve and I never have enough time together anymore. We both vowed that nothing would get in the way of our date. I had arranged for my parents to take the children for the weekend. I wanted the time to be romantic. I hoped we could get to know each other again.

"Over the past six months Steve's job had consumed him completely. On top of that, he spent a lot of time on rescue squad business. Miss a call? That's not Steve's nature. We needed some time together for the sake of our marriage.

"We were sitting in the restaurant. The soup had just been served. Suddenly 'Big Brother' spoke—his pager sounded. An auto accident. Steve looked at me and said, 'Sorry, honey, I have to go. I'll be right back.'

"I'm afraid people won't believe me if I tell them this story. But I'm sure other spouses of rescue and fire people can relate to it.

"OK, Steve returned to the restaurant in a half hour. But the damage was already done. I was angry and embarrassed. I felt abandoned. The night was over for me—and right then I felt our marriage was, too. We left the restaurant, picked up the kids, and went home.

"Why couldn't he understand? That night was important to me—to us. I remember saying to Steve, 'The next time I want to talk to you, I'm going to call 9-1-1 and threaten suicide. At least then I know I'll have your full attention.'"

Families and Stress

Pam's situation is not unusual. Up to now we've been talking mostly about the effects of emergency stress on the individual responder. But emergency service puts demands on families as well. In order to effectively cope with stress, you need to look continually at its impact on your family life. **Emergency service strains families.**

Statistics show a consistently higher rate of divorce among emergency responders compared to the general public. It's tragic that people who are motivated to help others frequently experience such a heavy burden in their personal lives. The sources of this strain are numerous:

- **Time demands.** For both career and volunteer responders, emergency activities claim a great deal of time out of a person's life. The hours are erratic. The tendency to give more and more time to emergency work is common.

- **Being "on call."** Just the potential to be called away for an emergency at any minute can strain a relationship. Knowing that their partners are ready to drop everything and rush to an emergency makes life difficult for emergency service spouses. And when it happens, as in the case of Steve and Pam, the sudden departure can damage a relationship.

- **Danger.** Emergency responders face dangers on even the most routine calls. Spouses and partners are the ones left behind to worry when responders go rushing off to a call. This type of worry can be stressful and wearing.

- **Negativity.** Emergency work puts us in contact with people who are in pain, seriously ill, injured, sometimes hostile. We see much that is depressing, including death. Sometimes we bring this negativity home. That puts another burden on our close relationships. Even if we don't talk about it, our partners can sense it's there.

- **Conflicting loyalties.** Who comes first, your family or your emergency colleagues? Most responders answer, "My family, of course." But in fact, there are often conflicting loyalties. Your spouse or your children may not always feel that your first loyalty is to them.

- **Emotional stress.** Few professions subject a person to the type of emotional stress that is a regular part of EMS work. The danger is that the responders will invest too much emotion in the job, leaving them drained and unresponsive at home. And if not properly handled, the stress that emotionally-charged emergencies generate can have an impact on many areas of your life, especially your close relationships.

The Result: Family Stress

The family stress that emergency service couples suffer is apparent in the frequent concerns they express about their lives:

"We don't have enough time for each other. What with work, raising kids, maintaining our home, attending drills, responding to calls, there's just no time left."

"We never talk. It seems like we're drifting farther and farther apart."

"The calendars and appointment books are always full. The pressure is constant. We never have time to relax and play as a family."

"I feel overwhelmed by responsibilities. I'm not getting any help from my spouse."

"We're always in a hurry. We never have time to relax."

"Sometimes I'd like to take that pager and throw it out the window."

Remember that it's not just your spouse who is affected by your emergency work. A woman whose father had been a fire service EMT said:

"I was always proud of my dad. I loved to go to the parades and picnics. But over the years I saw sadness in my father as well. He would come home from a midnight shift and Mom would say he was tired. But it was more than that. He'd been through something very difficult, an accident, or a death. It bothered him—I know that now. He couldn't just forget it. Whether he wanted to or not, he brought it home. We all shared his career, the good and the bad."

Your Family is Your Best Stress Defense

> *In all aspects of stress defense, it's helpful to have the support and encouragement of someone close to you.*

While emergency service can have a negative impact on your home life, your family can also be a very positive element in your effort to cope with daily stress. Isolation and feelings of loneliness make stress worse. Sitting down with your partner to talk about feelings, about the things you've experienced, helps you to cope.

In all aspects of stress defense, it's helpful to have the support and encouragement of someone close to you. You need someone who you can talk to without feeling inhibited. You need someone to discuss your plans and goals with. Often you need someone to help you maintain perspective, to remind you about what's really important.

You should work to prevent stress from damaging your relationships and at the same time try to take advantage of the very powerful contribution that your partner can make toward helping you cope with stress. This requires balance between your emergency work and home life. It requires, above all, regular communication with your partner.

The Six No's of Failed Relationships

1. No plans together
2. No interests together
3. No sharing
4. No contact
5. No communications

All add up to:

6. No hope

Question: How many No's currently exist in your relationship?

Keeping Secrets

"They don't understand." These three words sum up a whole range of problems that develop in emergency service families. Responders feel that their spouses don't really understand what it's like to do this kind of work. They don't know what it's like to work at a bad auto accident or a major structure fire. They don't understand the organization of the squad or department. They can't imagine the esprit de corps that develops among a group of rescuers. They have no idea of what that adrenaline rush is like, or of the type of letdown that can occur after a bad call. They simply don't understand.

"My wife just doesn't get what it's all about," a career paramedic told his marriage counselor. The therapist asked, "Have you tried to explain it, to help her understand?" The medic admitted, "No, I never have."

"The less they know the better," is the flip side of, "They don't understand." You deal with grim and emotionally powerful situations on a regular basis. You've decided that your partner doesn't want to know, would be better off not knowing. It would upset them. If you keep it from them, maybe it will be easier for you to deal with.

But the silent treatment doesn't prevent the stress of emergency service from infecting your relationship. The wife of the paramedic told the same counselor, "I *know* when he's had a bad day. I can see it and feel it."

Silence leaves your family wondering. Are you upset about a call, or about something they did? Is something seriously wrong? Is your mood related to work, or to some family issue? Without feedback your family members are likely to assume that your behavior is directed at them.

Here's what a group of spouses said during a group session following a line-of-duty death:

"Why can't they talk to us? Why can't they let us in on what's happened? Don't they think we know something's the matter?"

"Sometimes I'm not sure if I've done something wrong—or is it the job? When he's silent, I feel I'm in a guessing game with him. Is it me, the kids, or a bad call?"

"Tell them to talk to us. We won't crumble. How can we help, or be a support, a friend, or a wife, if they won't let us in. I don't need to understand the job to understand my husband's pain and sadness. I married him to be there in good times and bad. When he won't share his bad times with me he creates bad times for both of us. Together I think we can work anything through."

Remember once again that you are a Total Person. You cannot leave your emergency work completely behind you when you go off duty. You are bringing home the emotions. One day you might be sad because you've seen someone die. The next day you're flying because you've been able to save a life. Other days you're bored or frustrated or tense because of your work.

If you don't communicate, your family members don't know what to expect when you walk in the door. They see and feel the emotions without having any explanation for them.

The Importance of Communication

The solution is communication. And the important thing is what you communicate. Listen to the "war stories" that emergency people tell each other. They're almost always long on facts and short on feelings. They relate what happened, but little about how the person felt while it was happening.

The war stories you tell your spouse should be just the opposite. The gory details aren't important. Your spouse is not interested in the tension pneumothorax you diagnosed or the leaking cerebrospinal fluid. What's important to them is how you felt, how you feel now. That's the primary challenge when it comes to successfully balancing your emergency life with your family life. It's easy. All it takes is a few words:

"I had a bad call today. A guy, 42 years old, had a heart attack. He died in the ambulance."

"I went to an auto accident. It took us a long time to get the patients out of the car. I'm really beat."

"My captain criticized me in front of the squad for a mistake I made. I feel lousy."

"We had an emergency childbirth today. Everything went like clockwork. It's a great feeling."

It's easy, but it's hard. Talking about feelings does not come naturally for most emergency responders. We're stuck with The Superhuman Myth. We don't even recognize that we have emotions. But just as failure to express feelings creates stress in you, it creates stress in your family as well. It's time to start talking about it.

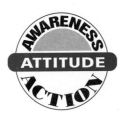

Awareness—

What am I keeping from my partner? What might my partner be wondering about? Have we ever sat down and talked about what emergency response is like?

Attitude—

"My partner is strong enough and tough enough to hear about both the good and the bad things about emergency service. For the sake of our relationship and my family, I'm going to be more open about the feelings that my work generates."

Action—

Put aside regular time to talk about how your day went. Maybe when you come home. Maybe after dinner when you've had a chance to unwind. Do it regularly. Don't wait for a bad call or a critical incident.

How To Be a Good Communicator

1. Accept what the other person is saying, don't immediately judge.

2. Summarize. Repeat back to them a summary of what they've said in order to make sure you understand and to let them know you're listening.

3. Pay attention to their feelings. Why they're saying something is as important as what they're saying.

4. Ask questions about facts. What happened to you today? How did your day go?

5. Ask questions about feelings. Did that make you feel bad? Do you ever get tired of that?

6. Hold the advice. Often your partner is talking just to let off steam. Don't jump in and tell them how to handle a situation.

7. Focus on the here and now. Dragging out past grievances often creates fruitless resentment. Don't save complaints to use as ammunition.

8. Don't argue in the bedroom. Don't go to bed without reaching some resolution of a disagreement.

9. Soften criticism with a compliment. A critical remark sandwiched between two bits of praise goes down much easier.

Keys to Effective Communication

Communicating with your partner is essential not just when it comes to balancing emergency work and family life, but in all areas of your relationship. It takes an effort. Talking is not necessarily communicating.

Start slow. Don't dive right into all the issues that have been troubling your relationship. Take some time to talk in general terms about what's been going on in both your lives.

Use a four-point process to address problems.
1. State what it is that bothers you.
2. State how it makes you feel.
3. Suggest a solution.
4. Invite comment.

Example: *"The other day when you weren't honest about where you went I felt betrayed. Next time, please trust me enough to tell me the truth. Don't you think that's a way to work this out?"*

Show your vulnerable side. Don't be afraid to say, "I need you." The tough-minded approach you take to your emergency work isn't the right way to relate to your partner.

Avoid the silent treatment. Silence is negative feedback. Silence shuts the door on communication. Always indicate to your partner that you are involved and paying attention. If you need time to think, say you do. Don't just clam up.

Don't rely on the "quick fix." To agree too readily to anything your partner says is a way of avoiding communication. Watch out for dismissive statements like, "Just don't worry about it," or "This will pass, you'll get over it." Remember, you won't always have the answer—problems cannot always be resolved instantly.

Avoid negative criticism. When talking about a difficulty, put the emphasis on how "I" feel about it, not on what "you" did. Don't get caught up in the blame game.

Choose the right environment. The wrong environment is in the family room with the television blaring and the kids screaming. The wrong time is after a bad call or when you're dead tired. Select a quiet time when you can sit down and look at each other. It's often good to get out of the house. Go for a walk together. Go to a movie and stop for dinner afterward.

Listen—really listen. We "listen" to television and the radio. But five minutes later, do we know what's been said? We monitor emergency radio traffic, but the messages for other units go in one ear and out the other. To really listen means to pay attention the way you do when an alarm sounds for your squad.

Active listening is work. You need to give the person your undivided attention. You need to suspend your judgments and assumptions until you genuinely understand what they're saying from their point of view.

You also need to pick up on nonverbal cues. Studies have shown that when people are talking together, only 7 percent of the total message that comes across is contained in the words. The tone of voice carries 38 percent of the message, and body language accounts for the rest, a full 55 percent. Keep in mind that it is not what you say, it's how you say it that causes the greatest impact on your listener.

> *It is not what you say, it's how you say it that causes the greatest impact on your listener.*

Validate your partner's feelings. If one person says, "This is important," and the other says, "No, it's not," you have the classic failure to communicate. Why? Because the second person is not validating what the first is saying. You have to recognize that your partner may be in a different space than you. They may have different concerns. Real communication requires you to acknowledge those concerns. A better answer is, "I hadn't given the matter much thought, but I see that it's important to you."

Talk about yourself. Good relationships are built on self-disclosure. Share your reactions to events. Take the risk of talking about your more secret feelings. It's the only way to forge a deep bond with your partner.

Say what you mean. Don't say, "I don't think we should go out tonight, you're tired," when you mean, "I'm beat." Dropping hints and speaking indirectly are not the best ways to communicate. Learn to come out and say, "This bothers me," or "I don't feel good when you do that," or "I'm angry about this."

A related communication problem is trying to "interpret" for the other person. "What you really mean is...." Making assumptions or jumping to conclusions are similar monkey wrenches in the machinery of communication.

Setting Priorities

In the story that opened this chapter, Steve is typical of emergency responders. He suffers from the 24/365 Syndrome—always ready to respond. Emergency work has taken over more and more of his life. He pays a price for this in terms of stress. But his spouse pays an equally serious price. Their marriage is in jeopardy.

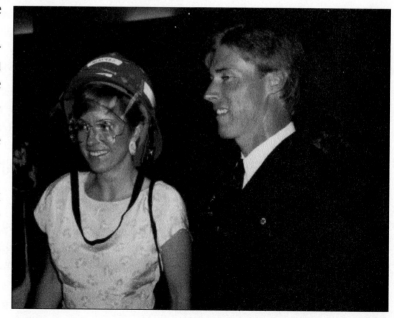

Emergency work can virtually take over your life. You become addicted to it. The squad, training, meetings, and calls all have top priority. Your marriage and family life come second. You put in more and more time on calls.

Emergency work can affect your life in many ways. Some of the changes will be positive and motivating, others will be negative.

Here are some of the signs that will be apparent to your spouse if your emergency duties are taking over in a negative way:

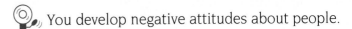 You develop negative attitudes about people.

You're more suspicious, more pessimistic.

You're less willing to socialize.

You talk less about your feelings.

You become rigid and authoritarian.

You criticize your spouse and kids excessively.

You're unwilling to admit mistakes.

You are developing the types of traits that lead to family problems. Those close to you become alienated. You become more distant and isolated, and the problem snowballs.

In practical terms, you only have so much time, so much energy. Emergency work requires an investment of substantial time, and of a great deal of both physical and emotional energy. Less and less remains available for your family.

Two additional dangers also affect emergency responders:

"Only what I do counts." They can fall into the trap of thinking that EMS work is so crucial that other roles, particularly the work their spouse does, are unimportant. This type of insensitivity is a powerful negative force in a relationship.

"Only my buddies can understand me." Another way emergency responders endanger relationships is to seek support only from other emergency people. Their colleagues have been there, they know what its like, they're easy to talk to. Another important aspect of the responder's life is removed from the home and transferred to the emergency service side.

Giving Time Back to your Family

One career EMS worker faced the problem of priorities head on:

"I've been working in emergency service for 20 years. There was a time when the work consumed me. I put in all the overtime I could get. I attended all the courses, read all the journals. What I didn't do was take time for me and my family.

"This went on for six years after I started work. Then one day my wife sat me down and started talking about a divorce. It hit me like a ton of bricks. I didn't even know we had a problem. I hadn't paid enough attention. But she sure knew.

"What's wrong? How could this happen? I was really at a loss. She said, 'You're never around. Your nose is always in some EMS text. It's all you ever talk about. You live for the ambulance business. You don't even know you have a family.'

"We needed help. We went for counseling. I did some serious thinking about my life. Now things are different. I'm still working in EMS, but I've balanced it with the rest of my life. I work my shift, keep current on the latest information, and leave time to enjoy my family. When I leave work, I leave the job behind as much as I can.

"I rediscovered the park. Now I find the time to play ball with my son. We all ride bikes in the evening. My wife and I go for a walk after dinner. It doesn't matter whether we talk or not, just being together is what counts. We even date again, go out for a movie and dinner.

"The best thing is that I've given up nothing, my job and EMS work are just as satisfying as ever. But spending time with my family has brought us all closer. It's something very valuable that I almost lost."

Take the time to include your family in your life. Block out time right now for family activities. Don't take the attitude that you'll finish everything else first, then spend what time is left with your family. Make family time your first priority.

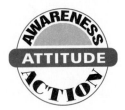

Awareness—

Take a close look at your priorities. Not what you think they are, but how much time you actually devote to the various aspects of your life. You may be surprised to find that family activities are well down on the list.

Attitude—

"Devoting time to the needs of my spouse and my children is as important as anything I do in my emergency work. I'm not going to allow that work to take over my life."

Action—

Learn to say no to the demands that are always taking you away from your family. Don't be afraid to say:

"Sorry, I can't do it. I'm playing ball with my kids."

"That's not a good time, I'll be at my daughter's play."

"I can't make it, my husband and I have plans."

"I won't be on call tomorrow night, I'm taking my wife to dinner."

Playing Together

One of the most effective antidotes to family stress is family fun. Play is a need we never outgrow. And it's important that families play together. Playing allows you to unwind and relax. It strengthens your relationship. It gets you out of your ordinary habits. It gives you the unstructured time together that you need.

Kids Feel Stress Too

Today more than ever, children are under stress. Drugs, divorce, school pressures, violence, all contribute to the pressures children feel. It's important to keep this in mind, and to help your kids use some of the techniques we've discussed to cope.

Be consistent with your kids. Help them to express their feelings and to keep things in perspective. Above all, take them seriously.

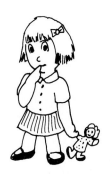

Play time is especially important for children. It's the easiest way to get involved in their lives and to relate to them in a positive way. Time goes by very quickly. Don't wake up someday to find that your kids are grown up and you missed spending time with them—you missed their childhood.

Easy games that involve everyone are ideal, things like volleyball, kickball, or croquet. The playful activities available are really unlimited. You can go with your family on a nature walk, fly kites, build sand castles at the beach, play cards, go bowling. Even work can be play; get the kids involved in raking leaves or digging the garden. The activity really isn't important—being together is.

Restoring the Couple

Think back to the time when you first met the person you're sharing your life with. Try to recall what it was like to be with that person—the excitement of going out, talking together, sharing every aspect of your lives. The hours together seemed like minutes—when you were apart all you could think of was getting together again.

Time Together

Take a survey of the time you spend with your spouse or partner during a typical week. How much time have you spent together?

Talking, with no one else around ...... _____

Looking at each other without talking .. _____

Having fun together without the kids
or anyone else .... _____

Making love .... _____

Planning for the future .... _____

Being together while each does other
things .... _____

Eating quietly together without
interruptions .... _____

Attending religious services, praying, or
contemplating .... _____

Total time together .... _____

Does the total amount of time that you invest in your relationship support your needs? Or does it reflect a neglect of your relationship? Relationships take work. Work takes time.

What happened? Life took over. Careers, activities, having kids, all the other aspects of life have gotten in the way. You have become more and more focused on the day-to-day things that need to be done, less and less focused on your relationship.

Emergency service work, whether as a career or in a volunteer capacity, places one more large burden on your time and attention. It's one more distraction away from that other person in your life.

As an EMS professional, you are courteous, polite, attentive and caring toward every person you deal with when you're responding to an emergency. What happens when you get home? How do you treat the person who is most important to you? Are you equally courteous and considerate? Or do you think, "I've had a long day, I can be myself now that I'm home?" Does being yourself mean feeling free to be rude and insensitive and self-centered?

Maybe you've come to take that person's love for granted. You feel it's OK to make demands because your partner understands you. So you act out behavior that you would never have dreamed of during the early days of your relationship. You act out behavior that would be unacceptable if you directed it toward your patients or toward the people you work with. Suddenly that person is "special" because you're especially rude to him or to her.

Couples who are in love and able to stay in love realize that the fireworks and magical feelings that occur during courtship will inevitably change. But to be successful over the long term, you must find a way to constantly renew your love, to transform the burst of romantic love into the deep day-to-day love that sustains relationships.

Six Tips For Couples

1. Make plans together. Looking at the future and where you're headed is the best way not to drift apart.

2. Be assertive. You each need to feel confident of your own territory. Learn to say no gracefully to each other.

3. Relax together. Get in the habit of taking walks together, exercising, or listening to music.

4. Laugh together. Humor is a great way to relieve the inevitable tensions.

5. Fight in a healthy way. Don't avoid disagreements. Air them without blowing up or attacking your partner personally. Afterward, reaffirm your love.

6. Plan time apart. Sometimes it's good to get away from each other for a while. A few days separation can help renew a relationship.

Examining Needs

A couple who had been married for 40 years came to a counselor. They'd been high school sweethearts and now they'd just become great grandparents. But their marriage was on the rocks.

After listening to a recitation of the many problems between them, the counselor asked, "Sally, what do you need from John?"

Sally thought for a minute and replied, "I'd like it if he'd just open the door for me."

It was a simple, concrete need. It was also symbolic of an attitude. John was surprised. "You never told me you wanted me to do that," he said.

When they left, John opened the door for his wife.

At their next counseling session, Sally explained, "My father always treated my mother with such courtesy. I thought John didn't love me any more, that he didn't care. But I see now that he just didn't know—because I never told him."

Forty years and she'd never really told him what she needed from him. She assumed, he assumed, and their marriage fell into danger.

You have to make your needs known. Needs that are not expressed will probably not be met.

This story is instructive because it emphasizes that you have to make your needs known. Needs that are not expressed probably will not be met. One of the most valuable tools you can develop toward building and maintaining a good relationship is expressing what's on your mind. Don't make your spouse guess.

EMS work brings special demands in this area. The wife of a career paramedic complained that her husband was frequently asked to hold over for another half-shift. He was eager to do so because of the extra money. She recognized that it was necessary. But he never called her. She would expect him home at a certain time, he wouldn't show up, she would worry.

"I always worry when he's at work anyway," she said. "I know there are a lot of risks. When he isn't home at the time he's supposed to be, I start to imagine all kinds of things. I expect the department chaplain to come to the door and give me the bad news. I can't help it."

Her need was simple: Let me know when you'll be late so I won't worry about you. But she never expressed it in those terms. She would nag and fight with him about it. He would omit calling her just to spite her. But once she explained the situation fully, her husband was happy to comply.

Keep these points in mind when expressing needs:

1. **It has to be a two-way street.** Each of you must tell the other what you need, what you expect.

2. **Keep the request positive.** Don't say, "You always ignore me," or "I can't stand it when you forget to call." Instead phrase it like, "It makes me feel good when you pay attention to me," or "I would worry a lot less if you called."

3. **Keep it specific.** Instead of asking your partner to *"listen more,"* you might request that they "save some time when I come home so that I can talk about how my day went."

4. **Don't pile on everything at once.** Focus on one need at a time so that the other person is not overwhelmed.

Intimacy and Romantic Love

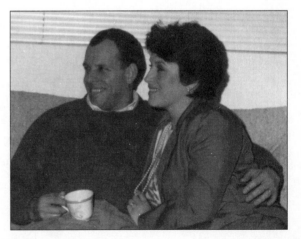

Intimacy means closeness. Two people can be close in physical, emotional, and mental ways. The word intimacy often evokes the physical or sexual aspect of a relationship. While physical intimacy is important, mental and emotional closeness are also crucial for couples. A satisfactory sex life does not guarantee these other forms of intimacy.

Emotional intimacy means expressing feelings openly. It means allowing your partner to express feelings and acknowledging those feelings. It requires you to put effort into understanding what your partner's emotional needs are, and fulfilling them whenever you can. Most important, it means not denying feelings—in yourself or in your partner.

Mental intimacy requires you and your partner to take time to engage in common interests. Certainly family, school and community issues, and the day-to-day management of your household will be interests that you have in common. Likewise you will share details about your respective jobs. But it's also very beneficial to develop additional interests together, whether it's sports, travel, gardening, cooking, theater or anything else.

Every successful relationship will include a lot of tender loving care. As an EMS provider, you know the value of TLC in emergency work—the Band-Aid that's not really needed, the hand you hold in the back of an ambulance. Your partner needs TLC every day. A touch, a hug, and all the little things that you can do that say, "You matter. I'm interested in you. I love you."

Restoring Romance

Emergency service is not conducive to romance. Difficult hours, intrusive interruptions, emotionally draining experiences, and simple fatigue all work against you. Building romance requires effort. You need imagination. You need to establish the right emotional climate.

Begin by getting rid of complacency in your relationship. Get out of the rut you've been in. Make an effort. Put in the time. Some of the elements of a romantic situation are:

- ❤ Freedom from distractions
- ❤ Dim lighting or candle light
- ❤ Walking in the moonlight
- ❤ Holding hands
- ❤ A quiet restaurant
- ❤ A picnic lunch in the park away from crowds
- ❤ Pleasant surprises
- ❤ Touching
- ❤ Gazing into each other's eyes
- ❤ A cozy winter night in front of the fireplace

All romantic situations include three elements:

Giving. It doesn't have to be a dozen roses. Often it's just giving the other person some of your time. Taking the time to cook them a dinner they especially like. Making the arrangements for a night out.

Surprise. Of course it's good to celebrate a birthday or anniversary. But it's even better to celebrate your relationship on no special occasion. Everyone loves surprises. They are the stuff of romance.

Sentiment. A child's crudely drawn "I love you" is worth more than the most expensive greeting card. Creating romance means not being afraid to be sentimental. Send your partner a love letter. Take them back to a place you used to go when you were dating.

At first you're bound to feel some embarrassment when you make the effort to create romantic situations. It may seem silly. But you'll find that your partner takes real pleasure in these situations, in the little things that you do. And romance can be like a breath of fresh air for your relationship.

Food For Thought

When was the last time you telephoned your spouse just to say, "I love you?"

How long has it been since you gave your spouse a small gift or did something to indicate "I'm thinking about you?"

In what specific ways do you demonstrate your support and encouragement?

When was the last time you planned a romantic evening with your spouse?

When did you last take time off from work simply to spend it with your spouse?

Balance, Commitment

The emergency work that you are doing is important. Your relationship with your partner is important. To succeed at both requires balance.

Your EMS work can create distance. There's the physical distance of long hours spent on calls, at drills, in training. There will also be emotional distance as you experience things that your partner will not fully share in. Sometimes you will be preoccupied or distressed because of events in the field. Things will come between you. That's inevitable.

To make your relationship work, you need a sense of commitment to each other. You need to let each other know that no matter what happens, you will support each other. You need to affirm that you are committed to your partner's goals, efforts, and growth, that you will be there when they succeed, and you will be there when they fail.

> **The growth, happiness, and long-term success of your relationship will depend on your ability to be open and honest, not to reject the other's needs.**

The growth, happiness, and long-term success of your relationship will depend on your ability to be open and honest, not to reject the other's needs.

All of this may seem difficult, and it is. A relationship is a success not because of magic, but because two people have worked to make it a success. Here are some comments from emergency service couples who have found the balance and commitment needed to sustain them over the years:

"I believe we have had a successful marriage because both of us have placed the relationship first in our lives. I think it's really a matter of priorities. Your relationship has to come above everything else. That doesn't mean that the ambulance squad can't be part of his life, only that it can't be his entire life."

"We talk about everything. We learned that when you hold it inside it never gets fixed. For 20 years it has worked for us. He even feels free to talk about the really bad, ugly calls he has responded to. He knows that I will listen and not judge him or what he did. It lets him get it out."

216

"We allow each other to grow in the areas we want. I love art—Tom really can't stand it. He loves the fire service—that's not for me. But we allow each other to pursue the thing that makes us happy. On occasion Tom will go with me to an art gallery. In turn, I have no problem attending some of his drill team events. In this small way we are able to share aspects of each other's life, while allowing each of us to fully participate in what we enjoy. Most important, we allow time for us as a couple. We never let our independent interests take all of our time."

"We have fun together. I know his ambulance work is serious. So is raising a family. I think we have kept it together because we have not lost track of the importance of having fun. We enjoy being together. The fun times balance the difficult times that every couple will experience. It's made the tough parts of marriage easier."

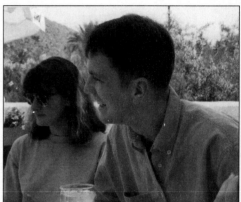

"We plan to be together. One thing we have learned is that if you don't make the plans, it won't happen. Everything else gets in the way. We set aside time for us, time to connect to each other. Sometimes it's only a few minutes to check with each other. Other times we actually have dates with each other. It's nice and it works."

"At least once a month we make a point of going to dinner and a movie with friends who are not connected with my work or with the ambulance."

"It takes courage to be in a good relationship. I've been married 32 years. I've lived through Larry being chief twice. It's taken a great deal of courage to remain committed. There were many times when our relationship suffered. We needed to adjust over and over. The thing that has seen us through has been the courage to confront misunderstandings, to say the things we feel, to admit when we're wrong, to trust each other."

SUMMARY

- Some of the aspects of emergency service that can have a negative impact on families are:
  Time demands
  Being "on call"
  Danger
  Negativity
  Conflicting loyalties
  Emotional stress

- The rescuer's family can also be their best defense against stress.

- Most emergency responders need to be more open with their partners—communication is essential.

- Effective communication requires you to choose the right environment, listen, validate your partner's feelings, say what you mean.

- The time you spend on emergency work compared to the time you spend dealing with family matters will indicate your real priorities.

- You need to devote unstructured time to your family, especially in the form of play.

- It takes real effort to make a relationship work.

- One key is for both partners to express in specific terms what they need from the other.

- Intimacy is not just physical closeness but includes emotional and mental aspects as well.

- Giving, creating surprises, and being sentimental are important elements in restoring romance to a relationship.

- Balance and commitment are the most important long-term elements in a successful relationship.

For Further Thought _____

1. What are the main aspects of emergency service that have the potential for damaging your relationships?

2. We know the symptoms of stress in an individual. What are some of the symptoms of stress in a family?

3. What are the things about emergency work that your spouse should know? What kind of things would they not want to know?

4. Why is it sometimes difficult to communicate with those close to us about the things that happen in EMS?

5. Good communication depends on the right time and place. What are some ways of creating situations in which communication can flourish in your family?

6. What are some good activities for putting play back into a relationship? How do these activities help keep a couple together?

7. Why is it important to express needs in specific terms?

8. Why is romance important in a relationship? Why is it often neglected?

9. What does intimacy mean to you?

10. What are some of the ways that emergency work can interfere with a fulfilling sex life?

CHAPTER 9

Living with an Emergency Responder: A Guide For Family Members

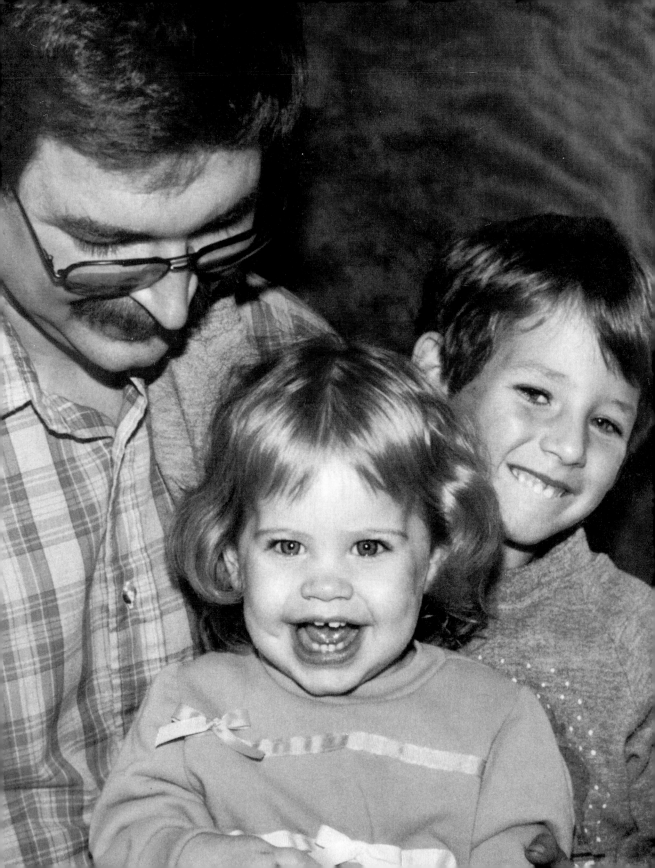

Living with an Emergency Responder: A Guide For Family Members

This chapter is for anyone who is living in a close relationship with an emergency responder. In many cases it will be a spouse or partner. The advice here may also be useful for the children, relatives and friends of emergency workers.

Emergency service spouses have often been neglected when it comes to considering the overall impact of stress. In fact, you are directly affected by the stress of your partner's job, and you are the person who can best help your partner to cope with that stress.

To be most effective, you need to move beyond a purely supportive role. You need to be active in maintaining your relationship, in helping your partner cope with the effects of stress, and in coping with the stress that you face yourself.

Strong relationships take work on the part of both partners. The information here will assist you to understand the nature of emergency service stress, and the effect it has on your loved one and on yourself. Utilize this material to strengthen and protect your relationship. It will also be useful for you to go over the material in Chapter 8.

Stress in Emergency Service

You're already aware that emergency work is stressful. You've seen your partner rush out to an auto accident in the middle of a winter night, or come home tired and depressed after a bad call. You probably know something of the difficult physical conditions in which your partner often works, the time pressures, the life-or-death decisions.

Stress is a normal reaction to events that are physically or emotionally demanding. Everyone has a capacity to adjust to stress. But sometimes the amount of stress or the special circumstances that a person is under prevent them from coping with pressures as they happen. In some ways, a person's system is like a rechargeable battery. As long has they have an opportunity to regularly absorb stress and regain their charge, they can keep going. But too many demands for too long can drain them until they have no more capacity to cope.

You need to keep two facts about stress in mind:

1. **Stress builds.** Often it's not any one thing that causes a stress reaction in an emergency responder. It's an accumulation of events, ranging from paperwork to major disasters. Stress can be insidious, building so slowly that a person isn't even aware of it. It can come from sources outside of emergency service as well. The daily stresses that we all encounter add more pressure to the serious stress of emergency work.

   You will often be the first to perceive that your partner is not coping with the accumulated stress. You will be the one to see the symptoms. You may be the one to sound the alarm that something is wrong.

2. **Stress spills over.** An emergency responder is a Total Person first, an EMT, paramedic or firefighter second. Each of us has various facets in our lives: physical, emotional, mental, social, and spiritual. Stress from one area can affect all the others. Stress in the emotional area can produce physical symptoms. Stress in a person's social life may show up as mental confusion or emotional instability.

Consider an example: If a relationship is in turmoil, each of the partners will experience powerful emotions. Those emotions will interfere with the person's ability to concentrate. They may cause sleep disturbances. Stress rarely remains confined to one realm.

224

The stress that an emergency worker experiences on the job is likely to affect all areas of his or her life. That's why you play a significant role in helping your partner to cope. Emergency stress can't be isolated. It's something that needs to be addressed by considering the Total Person. You are a big part of that person's life.

Just as stress spills over, the activities that defend against stress can take place in any of the areas of the person's life. Physical exercise, for example, is a great antidote to the mental stress that comes from having to pass a state qualifying exam. Social activities with friends can help alleviate stress that may be affecting a person's emotional life, and so on.

> *Emergency stress can't be isolated. It's something that needs to be addressed by considering the Total Person. You are a big part of that person's life.*

Who is the Emergency Responder?

Most emergency responders have a capacity to deal with stress successfully. They're resilient, tough-minded, flexible. They tend to be highly motivated. Their training and experience serves as a powerful buffer against stresses that would overwhelm most people.

They aren't, however, immune from the effects of stress. This is true no matter how long they've been on the job, no matter what grim sights they've seen in the field. Stress is an occupational hazard that never goes away.

Also, some of the positive traits of emergency responders make them more vulnerable to stress:

- They are good at keeping themselves and situations under control. This trait can work against them because they never express their emotions, they always want to be under control.

- They have high expectations. They always go into the field with the idea of getting the job done. But because they can't always be successful, their expectations sometimes create frustration and disappointment.

225

- They are detail-oriented, but sometimes the details of emergency work are very grim. It can be hard for them to erase grisly images from their minds.
- They love action. But much of emergency work—the training, waiting, routine calls—is tedious. Boredom can be stressful.

Think about how these traits apply to your partner. Talking over the ways in which they may lead to stress is an excellent form of early prevention.

Symptoms of Stress

Stress can produce a wide range of symptoms, from simple irritation to serious chest pains. Sometimes a person who is having trouble coping with stress will have many of the symptoms we associate with burnout—outbursts of anger, anxiety, complaints about being pressured.

But in many other cases the symptoms of stress are more subtle. The person may appear outwardly relaxed, but suffer from nightmares and frequent indigestion. The stress may show up in behavioral changes such as compulsive work or increased drinking. The person may be depressed, or may suffer frequent colds and other minor illnesses.

It's also not uncommon for the person to deny that they are suffering from stress. They may not perceive it themselves.

The main thing for you to consider is how their behavior or health has changed. If you detect significant changes in mood, behavior, or personality, you should consider that they may be having trouble coping with stress. In addition, here are some of the most common stress warning signs:

Sleep disturbances, particularly insomnia.

 Withdrawal. They don't want to be with friends anymore. They're often isolated.

 Fatigue. They don't have their usual energy.

 Apathy. They neglect themselves and the people around them. They just don't care anymore.

 Physical symptoms. Digestive problems, headaches, muscular pains, and many others.

It's important that you never dismiss any problem your partner is having as "just stress." The symptoms of stress are very real. They may also be a sign of an underlying physical problem that needs medical attention. If your partner experiences serious symptoms like chest pains and frequent headaches, urge them to visit a doctor as soon as possible.

Awareness, Attitude, and Action

We have used this AAA approach throughout the book. It represents a basic way of dealing with stress, and is one that you should urge your partner to take advantage of.

Awareness—

You can't take steps to cope with stress if you're oblivious to it. Awareness means stepping back in order to get some perspective on your life. It means frequently assessing yourself and your situation. Because stress is often hard to perceive directly, you can help your partner by encouraging periodic assessment.

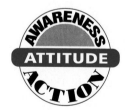

Attitude—

Once a person has become aware of the stress in their life, they need to realize that how they look at a situation is a big factor in the amount

of stress it causes. One person takes the attitude: "I am in control of my life, I'm not going
to let stress get the better of me." Another
thinks, "This situation is making me feel
stressed out and there's nothing I can do about
it." The first one is much more likely to cope
successfully.

Action—

The third step is crucial. The person has to do
something in order to keep stress from taking
over. Sometimes this means stress defense
actions: exercise, breathing, relaxation, social
activities. Other times it means doing something about the source of the stress: con-
fronting a demanding boss, getting household
finances in order, becoming better organized.

A Key Concept: Wellness

Health is a continuum. Illness is on one end, optimum
well-being on the other. Most of us spend our time somewhere in the middle. But stress tends to drag a person
toward the illness end. In order to live a healthy and balanced life, a person needs to take actions that move them
toward wellness.

Wellness does not refer only to freedom from illness. It
takes into account emotional, mental, and social well-
being too. It means having a sense of purpose in life, as
well as happiness, fulfillment and self-respect. All of these
aspects of life are interrelated.

There are four important things that you can encourage
your partner to do in order to keep moving toward
wellness:

1. **Accept change.** If a person is not coping with stress,
   some change is needed. Because change is hard in
   itself, we all tend to resist it. Recognize this and be
   supportive of the changes that your partner makes.

2. **Take action.** Procrastination, being stuck in a rut, feeling immobilized—these all add to stress. A person needs to do something in order to break the cycle of stress, in order to counteract the forces that move them away from wellness.

3. **Nourish yourself.** The body needs good food. The mind needs nourishment as well as interests and new knowledge. Learning new skills and having new experiences are antidotes to the effects of stress.

4. **Make choices.** You choose your life. Of course some things are beyond your control, but you choose how you react and what you do. To overcome stress a person has to take responsibility.

Supporting Your Partner

A person who is having trouble coping with stress must ultimately help himself or herself. You cannot do it for them, you cannot intervene directly. The best way to be useful is not to give them help, but to develop a helping relationship.

Here are a few things you can do:

Encourage communication. Ask questions: How did your day go? What was that call like? I'm interested if you want to talk about it.

One emergency service spouse asked her husband to describe exactly what he did during a day. The simple question elicited a full description of his day, including the many stressful events and issues he had to deal with. He was relieved to talk about it. She got a much better appreciation of what he had to face at work.

Listen without judging. Emergency responders are often sensitive to criticism. They have to make judgment calls regularly, and they resent having someone second-guess them. It's important that you remain neutral and supportive when you listen. Try to empathize with what your partner is feeling rather than make judgments about the facts of the matter.

Validate your partner's feelings. IT'S OK NOT TO BE OK. That's one of the most important messages you can pass on to your partner. It's OK to feel bad. It's OK to be afraid sometimes. It's normal. Let them know you understand. Stress tends to isolate. Having someone acknowledge what's troubling them helps a person to cope.

Express your confidence. Let your partner know that you feel they have the resources to handle stress, to make the changes needed in order to cope. Having someone believe in you is one of the strongest stress antidotes.

The Prince Charming Syndrome

Sometimes when problems arise in a relationship, a person is tempted to think they've chosen the wrong mate.

The point is not to find the right mate, but to be the right mate. Children, job changes, money problems, and emergency service work all require adjustments.

Instead of wishing for a mythical Prince or Princess Charming, try committing yourself to making the relationship work.

Avoid giving advice. Your partner will be quick to pick up on implied criticism. "Monday morning quarterbacks" are unwelcome in emergency service. Often we have an urge to give advice, to try to get actively involved in the problems of a loved one. But that suggests to the person that they aren't capable, they can't cope on their own. It's much better to let them know you trust their capacity to handle the situation and support the decisions they've made.

Time Together

Take a survey of the time you spend with your spouse or partner during a typical week. How much time have you spent together?

Talking, with no one else around . . . . . . _____

Looking at each other without talking . . _____

Having fun together without the kids
or anyone else . . . . _____

Making love . . . . _____

Planning for the future . . . . _____

Being together while each does other
things . . . . _____

Eating quietly together without
interruptions . . . . _____

Attending religious services, praying, or
contemplating . . . . _____

Total time together . . . . _____

Does the total amount of time that you invest in your relationship support your needs? Or does it reflect a neglect of your relationship? Relationships take work. Work takes time.

Suggest alternatives. Stress often creates "tunnel vision." The person becomes so focused on the problem, they can't see the solution. You can help by simply pointing out some of the possibilities. Don't express it in terms like, "Why don't you do this." Simply raise it as a possibility. Even better is to say something like, "When I feel that way, I do this."

Coping With Critical Incidents

Day-to-day cumulative stress is the most common problem for emergency responders. But sometimes a single incident will create so much stress that the person will be overwhelmed. This critical incident stress is a serious problem and one that you can help your partner to deal with.

First, it's important to keep in mind that a critical incident need not be a major disaster. A number of factors can turn a routine ambulance or fire call into a major stress factor. These include:

Trapped victims. It's very frustrating not to be able to provide care to a person immediately because he's trapped in a wrecked vehicle.

How To Be a Good Communicator

1. Accept what the other person is saying, don't immediately judge.

2. Summarize. Repeat back to them a summary of what they've said in order to make sure you understand and to let them know you're listening.

3. Pay attention to their feelings. Why they're saying something is as important as what they're saying.

4. Ask questions about facts. What happened to you today? How did your day go?

5. Ask questions about feelings. Did that make you feel bad? Do you ever get tired of that?

6. Hold the advice. Often your partner is talking just to let off steam. Don't jump in and tell them how to handle a situation.

7. Focus on the here and now. Dragging out past grievances often creates fruitless resentment. Don't save complaints to use as ammunition.

8. Don't argue in the bedroom. Don't go to bed without reaching some resolution of a disagreement.

9. Soften criticism with a compliment. A critical remark sandwiched between two bits of praise goes down much easier.

Incidents involving children. A sick or injured child almost always affects rescuers much more deeply than an adult patient.

Line-of-duty deaths. Besides losing a friend and colleague, a line-of-duty death is a grim reminder of every emergency responder's personal vulnerability.

Distraught relatives. Sometimes it's harder to deal with the extreme emotional reactions of bystanders than it is to handle the incident itself.

Another point to remember is that everyone reacts to events differently. A call that is a critical incident for one rescuer may be strictly routine for another. Often it's the accumulation of stress from other sources—difficult calls, long hours, financial problems—that make the person vulnerable to critical incident stress.

Critical Incident Stress is Normal

A person who has gone through a critical incident may experience noticeable symptoms. Flashbacks to the scene of the incident are common, as are vivid memories that just won't go away. The person may feel guilty for not having done more. They may be confused, emotionally numb, angry. They often withdraw from contact with others. Later symptoms can include loss of emotional control, depression, fatigue, inability to concentrate. These signs may be quite apparent to you even if your partner doesn't recognize them.

Your first task is to reassure your partner that what they are feeling is entirely normal. Sometimes these symptoms, especially the intrusive images of the incident, can be frightening. The person feels he is losing his mind. Or he's ashamed because he feels his reaction is a sign of weakness.

In fact, the symptoms of critical incident stress are a normal reaction to a powerful and unusual event. Even though all emergency responders, through their training and experience, develop psychological defenses against stress, anyone's defenses can be overwhelmed. And almost everyone who works in emergency service for any length of time can be affected by critical incident stress.

Talking is the Best Solution

The worst thing your partner can do when faced with critical incident stress is to try to "tough it out." Studies have shown that even if the person is able to suppress the immediate effects, they may be subject to delayed stress, the symptoms of which include behavioral and emotional changes, such as intense irritability and vivid nightmares.

The best way to avoid long-term problems is for the person to talk about the event and about their reactions and feelings.

The best way to avoid long-term problems is for the person to talk about the event and about their reactions and feelings. This gives them an opportunity to let out the emotions and thoughts they've been holding inside. It also provides a chance to reassure them that what they're feeling is normal, that others feel the same thing, that their reaction to the event is not an indication of weakness or mental illness.

Many agencies have established formal critical incident stress debriefing (CISD) programs in which all the rescuers who respond to a disaster are called together a few days later to talk about the incident under the guidance of a mental health professional and several peer counselors. These programs have proven to be very effective. You should encourage your partner to attend.

When CISD is not available or appropriate you can help your partner by encouraging them to talk about the incident that's bothering them. Here are some hints for doing this effectively:

1. **Wait a day or two.** Don't try to get the person to talk immediately after the incident. They need a while to absorb what's happened and to sort out their feelings.

2. **Start with what happened.** Don't question them about their feelings right away. These things are hard to talk about. First get them to describe what they did and saw at the incident.

3. **Never judge.** The person may blame himself, or may be angry or remorseful. You should remain neutral and supportive. Don't criticize, don't offer advice. Just listen.

4. **Encourage communication.** Ask questions that draw the person out: "Tell me more about that." "Tell me what you mean." "What was it like for you?" Provide plenty of nonverbal support by maintaining eye contact and frequently touching your partner.

5. **Know your limits.** If you feel the assistance of a mental health professional is needed, urge your partner to obtain that help. Reassure them that it's the wise and understandable course to take. Try to determine whether the person is making progress in dealing with the incident, or whether the problem is getting worse. Continued depression, isolation, sleeplessness, agitation, alcohol abuse, or any talk of suicide should alert you to the need for immediate counseling.

Support for Families

Spouses and other family members can often benefit from a formal debriefing process after a critical incident. This is especially true in the case of a line-of-duty death. Many CISD teams now arrange for such debriefing sessions. Find out about the services offered in your area.

In addition, support groups that allow the families of emergency responders to exchange information and encouragement can be found in many places. These groups can be a useful way to deal with both day-to-day stress and critical incidents.

The Road to a Better Relationship

You already know that emergency service can put a burden on a relationship. It consumes your partner's time and energy, it affects their moods, it can interrupt activities you plan together. One of the most serious consequences of emergency service stress is the way in which it erodes relationships.

The continuum of wellness might be applied to the well-being of couples, too. The combined stresses of emergency work and daily life continually push the relationship toward difficulties. In order to counteract this effect, you both need to do those things that renew and invigorate your feelings for each other.

Here are 10 suggestions for doing so:

1. **Guard your time together**. It's too easy to become ships passing in the night. If you don't make specific efforts to spend time together, the demands of family, job, community activities and emergency service will eventually eat up all of your time. You need to realize that the time you spend with your partner, talking or just being together, is one of your highest priorities. Don't let other things interfere. Learn to say no to the demands that cut into this time.

2. **Maintain a social network.** It's important for emergency responders to have friends outside the ambulance squad or fire department. While it's great to attend social events with your partner's colleagues, you should make sure that both of you make and maintain friendships among a broader circle. Having friends to talk to and support you is a crucial stress defense, and you need to make those friends in advance of a crisis.

3. **Laugh together.** EMS work is often a grim business. Emergency responders need to take time to look at the lighter side of life. Encourage your partner to get out to see a comic movie, to visit an amusement

park, or to engage in other light-hearted activities. Share jokes and funny stories. Learn to laugh about life's minor setbacks.

4. **Touch often.** A hug, a kiss, a squeeze of the hand, an arm over the shoulder, all of these are potent antidotes to the tension that stress creates. Touching is a powerful form of nonverbal communication. An absence of physical contact can be a warning sign that stress is taking over.

5. **Exercise together.** Exercise is both an excellent stress remedy and a good way for the two of you to spend time together. The simplest approach is simply to take a walk together every day. You not only burn off calories, you have a convenient time to talk to each other.

6. **Compliment your partner.** Emergency service people are often quite modest about their accomplishments. They save a life, but insist that they're simply doing their job. Unfortunately, they usually receive a minimum amount of gratitude or recognition for what they do. Let your partner know that you appreciate their contributions, that you are proud of them and recognize the courage and dedication that emergency work requires. It's a message you can't repeat too often.

7. **Say what you mean.** Speak to your partner directly. Use words like:

"I feel rejected when you do that."

"I like it when you are that way."

"It makes me angry when you do that."

"I'm afraid when you don't communicate with me."

Let the person know what you need and want and feel. If there are issues that you think need to be talked about, come right out and put them on the table. Don't hint or insinuate.

8. **Learn the art of compromise.** For anyone to incorporate emergency work into their life, continual trade-offs are necessary. Instead of making all-or-nothing demands, you should try to resolve conflict through compromise.

   "I don't mind the time you're putting into your EMT course, but let's take a long weekend together when it's over." "It's OK for your squad members to call here about problems, but let's limit the hours."

9. **Put things in proportion.** Sometimes your partner will begin to get the idea that emergency work is the only thing that's important. You can provide valuable perspective by reminding them of the other things in life—marriage, children, personal development.

   You might remind your partner of the first rule of stress management: Don't sweat the small stuff. Stress often makes a person become so focused on minor difficulties that they lose all perspective. At these times, it's very helpful to have someone who can say, "Wait a minute. Let's look at this. What's really important here? What's going to seem important five years from now?"

10. **Give your partner space.** It's important to emphasize that you can only do so much to help your partner deal with stress. Sometimes, all you can do is allow them to resolve the problem themselves. In any case, they need to have the time and space necessary to cope with day-to-day stress. This may mean time alone to unwind and relax after a hard day.

Set Goals Together

When you are eagerly looking forward to something, problems that would otherwise bother you seem much less important. One of the best ways to combat stress is to work toward specific goals. It gives your life a purpose and keeps you from becoming obsessed with the trivial irritations that beset you.

The same is true for couples. Those who work together to achieve their objectives tend to be happier and less subject to stress. It's a good idea to regularly sit down with your partner and talk about where you are headed individually and as a couple. Make plans and talk about the timetable for achieving the goals.

Your planning should include all areas of your life, including work, leisure, health, financial, and social.

Make sure your plans are realistic, not pie in the sky.

Break long-term goals into intermediate and short-term goals that you can take action toward immediately.

Talk about the role each of you will play in making the plans a reality.

Take the attitude that your life together is an adventure.

Six Tips For Couples

1. Make plans together. Looking at the future and where you're headed is the best way not to drift apart.

2. Be assertive. You each need to feel confident of your own territory. Learn to say no gracefully to each other.

3. Relax together. Get in the habit of taking walks together, exercising, or listening to music.

4. Laugh together. Humor is a great way to relieve inevitable tensions.

5. Fight in a healthy way. Don't avoid disagreements. Air them without blowing up or attacking your partner personally. Afterward, reaffirm your love.

6. Plan time apart. Sometimes it's good to get away from each other for a while. A few days separation can help renew a relationship.

Take Care of Yourself

In order to help your partner cope with stress, you need to take specific actions to deal with the effects of stress yourself. In addition to the stressful events of daily life that we are all subject to, you have the additional burden of knowing that your partner is involved in a dangerous job that's often wrought with negativity.

You also need to make efforts to move toward wellness in the various facets of your life. You need to keep aware of the effects stress might be having on you, and adjust your attitude so that you aren't compounding the stress by blowing things out of proportion.

Here are some suggestions:

Be assertive. Remember that you are in control of how you respond to the events of your life. No one "makes" you do anything or feel a particular way. It's your decision. Know when to say no to demands or to another's interpretation of events.

Don't worry. Shut off those thoughts that keep recycling though your mind. Just say aloud or to yourself: Stop! Worrying does no good, it wastes energy, and it leaves you stressed.

Arrange for quiet time. Don't fill your schedule to the extent that you have no time for yourself. Every day you need to be alone and have at least a short period of time to think and reflect.

Exercise regularly. Walk, swim, jog, or ride a bike. Do something you enjoy. It keeps you fit and is a great stress defense.

Relax. Take a hot bath, lie down and listen to music, shut yourself in a room and read a good book. Any form of physical relaxation is helpful for combating the tensions that build during the day. Make it a habit.

Eat well. Make sure you eat a balanced diet. Everyone who is frequently under stress needs plenty of vitamin C, calcium, and the B-complex vitamins.

Spend time with friends. Social support is an effective defense against daily pressures. But when you feel stressed avoid those friends who are negative or demanding.

Breathe deeply. Deep breathing tends to ease stress—tight, restricted breathing makes it worse. Whenever you feel pressured, stop and take a few slow, deep breaths.

SUMMARY

The stress that effects emergency service people often builds over time.

- Stress can affect all areas of a person's life: social, emotional, mental, physical, and spiritual.

- The traits that make people successful emergency responders can also work against them by contributing to stress.

- The symptoms of stress can show up in many areas, but the person suffering from stress will not necessarily appear or feel pressured.

- Awareness, attitude and action are three key ways to approach stress management.

- The idea of wellness requires a person to do things to counteract the negative forces that contribute to stress and illness.

- You can support someone who is subject to emergency service stress by expressing your confidence in their ability to cope, encouraging communication, listening to them, and validating their feelings.

- Critical incidents can be occasions of overwhelming stress.

- The best way for the rescuer to deal with stress is to talk about what happened and about what they feel.

- Relationships succeed because both parties work at them.

- Planning and setting goals together is a good way to maintain a sense of purpose and to turn life into an adventure.

- Partners of emergency service people need to take care of themselves in order to deal with everyday stress.

For Further Thought ——————————

1. Why does an emergency responder need to be concerned about the stress of daily life in addition to the pressure from emergency situations?

2. List some of the signals of stress you've learned to recognize in your partner.

3. How do the ideas of awareness, attitude and action apply to some of the stresses that each of us faces every day?

4. Why is prevention a key component in the concept of wellness?

5. Communication is an important part of dealing with stress. But your partner doesn't want to talk about their feelings or the pressures they're under. What can you do?

6. Why might your partner be reluctant to discuss the emergency incidents that affect them the most?

7. One of the ways in which emergency work can damage a relationship is to use up the time that a couple could otherwise spend with each other. What are three ways to make sure you have enough time together?

8. What are the tactics that have already worked for you to renew your relationship?

9. What activities can you participate in with your partner that will help both of you to defend against stress?

The
10 Commandments
of Stress
Management

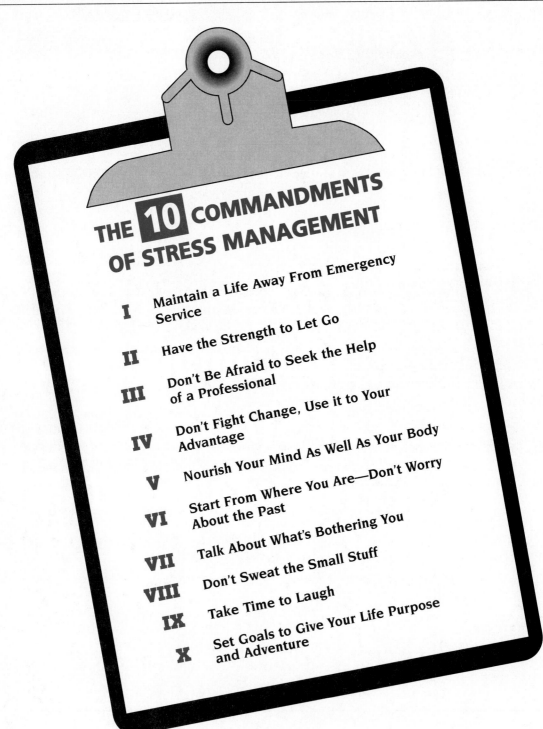

THE 10 COMMANDMENTS OF STRESS MANAGEMENT

I	Maintain a Life Away From Emergency Service
II	Have the Strength to Let Go
III	Don't Be Afraid to Seek the Help of a Professional
IV	Don't Fight Change, Use it to Your Advantage
V	Nourish Your Mind As Well As Your Body
VI	Start From Where You Are—Don't Worry About the Past
VII	Talk About What's Bothering You
VIII	Don't Sweat the Small Stuff
IX	Take Time to Laugh
X	Set Goals to Give Your Life Purpose and Adventure

The 10 Commandments of Stress Management

They'd gone through more than 100 hours of lectures together. They'd practiced their skills, they'd read the books, they'd agonized over the tests. Now the EMT class was over and they were walking outside after having completed the written state qualifying exam.

One member of the group turned to his friends and said, "Now we can start to forget it all."

He was joking, but he also had a point. We all know how the pressures we encounter in the field sometimes make it hard to apply all the details that seemed so clear in class. Situations that are simple in theory can be much more complicated in practice.

You will find the same thing when you begin to apply what you've learned in this book to the stress you encounter in your emergency work and in your life. Coping with the problem of stress can be a complicated, difficult, and sometimes frustrating task. Just when you thought you had everything under control, new problems arise.

The way to be successful in handling stress is the same way you are able to maintain your EMT skills: by continually refreshing, continually learning. Stress management is not a one-time effort. It's a lifetime project.

There are several important guidelines you can take away from this book.

Awareness, Attitude, Action

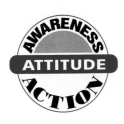

Be aware of the stresses in your life and what they are doing to you.

Adopt the attitude that you can cope, you can handle the pressure you're under.

Take action to defend against stress and to deal with the stress at its source.

A Lifestyle of Wellness

Do things now that will move you toward increasing well-being. Don't wait until stress drags you toward the illness end of the spectrum.

Consider Your Total Person

Pay attention to the stresses and challenges in all parts of your life. Always keep in mind that under your uniform you are a Total Person, with physical, mental, emotional, social, and spiritual needs.

The 10 Commandments

You've seen them throughout the book. Now you understand what they mean. It's a good idea to review them frequently. They should serve as a way to remember the basic concepts of emergency stress management.

I Maintain a Life Away From Emergency Service

Don't let your emergency work soak up all of your time, your attention, or your energy. Get a life.

II Have the Strength to Let Go

At times it really does require courage to face the difficult and powerful emotions inside you.

III Don't Be Afraid to Seek the Help of a Professional

You wouldn't advise a person with a broken arm to try to fix it on his own. When it's needed, professional help is simply the smart way to go.

IV Don't Fight Change, Use it to Your Advantage

The dinosaurs didn't change—they became extinct. You deserve a better fate.

V Nourish Your Mind As Well As Your Body

Keep growing, keep inquiring, keep caring.

VI Start From Where You Are—Don't Worry About the Past

Yesterday's a cancelled check. Tomorrow's a promissory note. Today's the only time you have. Spend it wisely.

VII Talk About What's Bothering You

Talk about it and let it go. It's not always easy, but it's the only way to keep issues from festering.

VIII Don't Sweat the Small Stuff

What's really important? How will you see this five years from now?

IX Take Time to Laugh

There is humor in the world around you. All you have to do is find it.

X Set Goals to Give Your Life Purpose and Adventure

Your life can be an adventure. And while every adventure has its obstacles, your sense of purpose will help you to overcome them.

The Choice is Yours

The challenges faced by emergency service people are increasing every day. Think about the training demands, the legal threats, the risk of AIDS, the problem of violence. It's not an easy job that you've chosen.

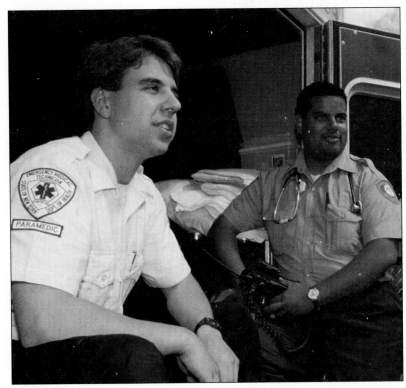

Stress is a fact of life. Even if you apply every technique in this book, you will still face the challenge of stress. There's no magic wand that can make it go away.

The question is whether you are going to effectively cope with the inevitable stress that will come your way, or whether you will allow stress to end your emergency service career. The threat is real. Emergency responders are dropping out of the field every day because they can't find a way to deal with stress.

Handling stress effectively requires commitment, not wishful thinking. It requires a life-long process, not a short-term program. It requires the same type of courage and dedication that you have already demonstrated in your work.

You can decide to cope effectively with stress. If you do so, you can look forward to a productive and satisfying career. If you decide to ignore stress or give in to it, then you face a difficult road ahead.

The choice is yours.

Resource Appendix ────────────

For information on stress management and intervention services or CISD teams in your area, contact your state EMS office. This number can be found in the state government listings of most telephone books. The state EMS office will also know if your state is a part of the Critical Incident Stress Management (CISM) Network.

Additional listings of state resources can be found in the reference book, *Medical 911*, published by Jems Communications.

The International Critical Incident Stress Foundation (ICISF) provides CISD education and support services to emergency services personnel and organizations. A list of books and videos on stress and emergency services related topics can also be obtained from the ICISF.

ICISF
5018 Dorsey Hall Drive, Suite 104
Ellicott City, MD 21042
410/730-4311
Fax: 410/730-4313
Jeffrey T. Mitchell, Ph.D., President
George S. Everly Jr., Ph.D., Chairman

The following individuals are active in various areas of stress management for emergency responders and their families. Use the information below to request specific information on resources available to you, your family, and your organization.

AK	Denny Patella, LCSW 907/561-2868
AZ	Tom McSherry, Former Chairman, Arizona CISM 602/267-4109
CA	Dan Costello, Fire Captain, CISD Coordinator 916/538-6849
	Mauguarite Jordan, RN, MPA 213/881-2485
	Barbara Massey, RN, NP, MS 213/738-4813
	Robert T. Scott, Ph.D. 818/995-3168
	Bonnita Wirth, Ph.D. 818/796-3515
CT	Guy J. Schiller, MA, CAC 203/233-6228
	JoAnne K. Supple, BA 203/576-6000
DE	Joe Rykaczewski, Fire Chief 302/998-8829
HI	Ana Horne 808/971-2508
IL	Carolyn Burns, RN, MSN, CS 708/474-6610

IN   Glen C. Calkins, Executive Director CISD-IN
800/382-9922

Lindi Kempfer, MS, EMT-P
317/929-3327

MD   Diana Schofield, LCSW (Military)
703/696-2066

Gregory Valcourt, NREMT-P
202/673-3234

Victor Welzant
410/828-0761

MN   Daniel L. Casey, MA
612/743-3581

Charles G. Cook, LSW
612/458-5277

NE   M. Thomas Perkins, Ph.D., ACSW
308/635-3171
308/632-5549

NJ   Raymond F. Hanbury Jr., Ph.D.
908/223-6849

Jakob Steinberg, Ph.D., ABMP
201/593-8556
201/586-8770

NY   Grady Bray, Ph.D.
315/536-0849

William F. Meehan
518/639-8888

Douglas J. Mitchell, MPA, Lt. NYC Fire Department
212/860-9268

Edward H. Sharrow, Co-Coordinator Upstate NY CISD
800/925-0956

Ray Shelton, Ph.D., EMT-CC
516/681-3976

OH   J.R. (Bob) Gribble, Battalion Chief
216/881-2473

PA   Kay Carman, Field Coordinator
717/843-5111

Lynn Kennedy Ewing, Delaware County
   CISD Coordinator
610/565-9575

RaeAnn Fuller, RN, EMT-P
708/356-9918

RI   B. Anne Balboni
401/467-3377

TX   Paul A. Tabor, MS, EMT-P, State CISM Coordinator
512/834-6749

VA   Chip Theodore
703/204-3386

WA   Linda Ott, MSW
509/926-6699 (pager)

CANADA   Leigh Blaney, Clinical Coordinator, North Island
   CISM Society
Campbell River, British Columbia
604/339-3010

Murray N. Firth, B.M.C.A.
Barrie, Ontario
705/739-6226

David Jensen
Calgary, Alberta
403/273-5897

Garry Norris, MSW
Kenora, Ontario
807/468-6099

Reading List ──────────────

1. Brallier, L. *Successfully Managing Stress*. National Nursing Review, 1982.

2. Charlesworth, E. and Nathan, R. *Stress Management— A Comprehensive Guide to Wellness*. Atheneum, 1984.

3. Chernin, D. and Manteuffel, G. *Health: A Holistic Approach*. Theosophical Publishing House, 1984.

4. Davis, M., McKay, M. and Eshelman, E. *The Relaxation and Stress Reduction Workbook, 2nd ed.* New Harbinger Publications, 1983.

5. Girdano, D.A. and Everly G.S. *Controlling Stress and Tension: A Holistic Approach*. Prentice-Hall, 1986.

6. Hafen, B., Frandsen, K., Karren, K. and Hooker, K. *The Health Effects of Attitudes, Emotions, Relationships*. EMS Associates, 1992.

7. Lerner, H. *Stress Breakers*. CompCare, 1985.

8. Lovelace, T. *Stress Master*. John Wiley & Sons, 1990.

9. Mitchell, J.T. and Bray, G. *Emergency Services Stress*. Brady, 1990.

10. Peale, N. *The Power of Positive Thinking*. Center for Positive Thinking, 1990.

11. Selye, H. *The Stress of Life*. Free Press, 1956.

12. Tubesing, D. *Kicking Your Stress Habits*. Whole Person Associates, 1985.

About The Authors

Ray Shelton, Ph.D., EMT-CC, is an educator, mental health counselor, trainer, and consultant specializing in wellness and stress management in emergency workers and their families. Dr. Shelton has more than 30 years of field experience in emergency service as both a volunteer firefighter and an advanced ambulance medical technician with the Nassau County (N.Y.) Police Department. He is the supervisor of all EMS training at the Nassau County Police Academy, as well as an adjunct faculty member at Suffolk County Community College in the EMS training program. Dr. Shelton holds certifications as an advanced EMT instructor and as a master police instructor. He is the clinical director for both the Nassau County and Suffolk County Critical Incident Stress Debriefing programs. He lectures nationally to a wide variety of audiences on the subjects of stress and wellness. He is the author and presenter of a video training program titled, *Managing* EMS *Stress Through Wellness*, and has authored numerous articles on wellness. Dr. Shelton holds a master's degree in counseling psychology and a Ph.D. in health and human development.

Jack Kelly, EMT, is the author of 12 nonfiction books and numerous articles. He is a member of the Milan (N.Y.) Rescue Squad.